RYAN P. SHERMAN, DBH, KATY CABBAGE, PHD

WEIGHT LOST

WEIGHT LOSS PLAN

GAP ANALYSIS

IDEAL WELLNESS VISION

PERSONAL VALUES

SELF-ASSESSMENT

5 STEPS
TO ACHIEVING
YOUR **IDEAL WEIGHT**
AND **GAINING THE LIFE**
YOU'VE ALWAYS
WANTED

WEIGHT
LOST

*5 Steps To Achieving Your Ideal Weight and
Gaining the Life You've Always Wanted*

Ryan P. Sherman, DBH
Katy Cabbage, PHD

START HERE

We couldn't fit all of the resources you'll need to create an effective and sustainable weight loss plan into this book, as much as we wanted to. But we did create a webpage that offers all of our resources to readers for free. To maximize your weight loss results, we recommend downloading at least the first two resources before you start reading.

Resources

Weight Lost Self-Assessment: https://weightlostacademy.com/free-weight-lost-self-assessment/

Weight Lost Planning Template:
https://weightlostacademy.com/weight-lost-planning-template/

Weight Lost Blog: https://weightlostacademy.com/blog/

Weight Lost Satiating Meal Design Guide:
https://weightlostacademy.com/weight-lost-satiating-meal-design-guide/

Weight Lost High Protein and Fiber Breakfast Recipe Guide:
https://weightlostacademy.com/high-protein-and-fiber-breakfast-recipes/

Weight Lost Website: https://weightlostacademy.com/

Table of Contents

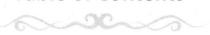

Phase Two: Explore

Phase Three: Create and Lunch

Introduction

Nobody Wants to Be Told What to Do

December 21, 2012

It's just a few days before Christmas, and I'm looking outside my tenth story office window at Massachusetts General Hospital (MGH) watching snowflakes swirl around the tightly packed high-rises in Boston's West End. All week long, gifts, flowers, and food (so much food) have been dropped off in droves by thankful patients to the primary care practice I work in. These generous patients have been expressing their gratitude for the entirety of the holiday season by arriving with care packages in hand, smiles on their faces, and a hug ready for each one of my colleagues, physicians, nurses, secretaries, and medical assistants. Watching these caring exchanges take place, I can't help but wonder, what about me? Where are all of my patients? As their health coach, I've formed strong relationships with nearly every one of my patients, and I have supported them so that they could significantly improve their health. Some of my patients have even lost more than 100 pounds. So, where are my card and my cookies? I like cookies!

In my previous job at Boston Medical Center, I was frequently showered with gifts and admiration, especially around the holidays. So why should this year be any different? I'm still the same nice guy.

1

Well, what I didn't realize while I was watching the snowflakes dance around the evening sky, pining for a holiday sweet that was baked in my honor, was that things were actually completely different.

My patients at Boston Medical Center, by my own doing, needed me, no, relied on me to improve their health. However, by helping my patients at MGH design their own plan to improve their health, which was most often a weight-loss plan, I had helped instill within them a strong sense of self-efficacy. As a result, their weight-loss plans worked and kept working long after they had left my care, which, of course, brought me great satisfaction. But because of this approach, my patients didn't view my role, which was to help them to create their own successful weight-loss plan, as something that they should be thanking me for. And you know what? They were absolutely correct. They were the ones who created and executed the plan; I was just the facilitator. Do you know what facilitators don't receive the week before Christmas? They don't receive holiday hugs, and they definitely don't receive cookies. Lucky for me, my colleagues at MGH were terrific at sharing.

Before leaving for the day, I grabbed a large chocolate chip cookie, which I planned to enjoy on my train ride home, and headed for the door. During my one mile walk to South Station to jump on the commuter rail home, I had time to think about how pretty the city was this time of year, covered in Christmas lights and a thin dusting of snow. But I spent most of my walk reflecting on the many patient success stories I had witnessed this past year and how I didn't expect any of these patients to return to my care since they now knew how to create sustainable behavior changes them to maintain their ideal weight. After weaving my way through the busy station, I spotted my train, and as I strode toward it, I paused in front of a large metal trash can and took the cookie out of my bag. As I let the cookie sail toward the barrel, I thought about how proud I was of my patients and how the connection I have built with them had led to the exact type of relationship I had dreamed of having with them when I started my work at MGH eighteen months ago.

How to Avoid Short-Lived Weight Loss and Long-Term Frustration

If I were to ask you the most critical elements of a successful and sustainable weight-loss plan, you'd probably reply "diet and exercise." This is certainly not a horrible answer by any definition, and these are generally behaviors that need to shift for weight loss to occur. However, from the research I have conducted, and from the experiences of the hundreds of patients I have worked with, I have realized that a person must do two things really well to lose a lot of weight and keep it off for good: create their own weight-loss plan and periodically set goals/reflect on their progress. Without these two elements, a person might lose weight, even a lot of weight for a short period of time, but those lost pounds are inevitably likely to return, and then some. This cycle of short-term success followed by gaining the weight back can be frustrating and even demoralizing, which is why this book is going to help you learn how to apply a much different approach to weight loss, an approach that is focused on supporting you to create and execute a weight-loss plan that allows you to attain a weight that makes you feel your best and to maintain that weight for as long as you so desire. But before you begin your journey toward your ideal weight, let's take a moment to understand better why trendy programs, fad diets, and even expert advice can only deliver weight-loss shortcuts that yield very temporary results.

In the United States, the weight-loss market is big business, having a total worth of over $70 million. New weight-loss programs are constantly being churned out to compete in such a vast marketplace and fuel industry growth. In fact, almost anytime I turn on the TV, open a webpage, watch a video on YouTube or scroll through my Instagram account, I am exposed to some sort of new weight-loss program or fad diet. This barrage of ideas, which often claim to be based on "science" and almost always are associated with a personal success story of someone who lost a large amount of weight in a very short period of time by following this program, can leave the consumer overwhelmed and thoroughly confused about what approach will actually work for them.

Almost all of these programs or products are designed to yield short-term, eye-popping weight loss results. I'm sure you've heard terms like "lose 10 pounds in the first ten days or get your money back" or "lose 15 pounds in seven days with . . . " What you never hear about is what happens after you lose that initial weight. Are people able to sustain this weight loss? Do most people just gain the weight right back? Well, the truth is that nearly all of these weight-loss programs are designed to help you achieve short-term, unsustainable results so that they can keep you engaged with their product or platform for as long as possible, and they are able to accomplish this by making you reliant on their services.

Weight-loss programs that yield short-term results by telling you exactly what path to follow or, in some cases, actually doing the leg work for you, come in many shapes and sizes and are a dime a dozen. The simplest example of this type of weight-loss plan is the fad diet. A fad diet promises unreasonably fast weight-loss results and is usually popular for a short period of time. While I'm writing this, the Keto Diet is the current flavor of the month, but not long ago, juice pressing was quite popular, and before that, the "Peel-a-Pound Soup" was a bit of a thing. These examples have elements of a comprehensive weight-loss strategy, but they typically inflate just one of these components to produce quick but unsustainable results. The more complex and more expensive weight-loss plans combine several of these elements into a packaged program that is designed to keep you engaged with their products.

Some of the major players in the weight-loss industry have created programs that DO produce weight-loss results but DO NOT help you sustain these results on your own. These types of programs will often send you several meals and/or shakes to consume a day. And guess what? If you eat only the food they send you/instruct you to eat, you'll lose weight because they decide what type of food and how much of it you can eat. So what happens when you want to go out to eat with your friends, or you simply get tired of paying through the nose for their pre-packaged foods? Well, when you reach this point (and you will reach this point), you most likely will gain the weight back, feel the desire to lose it again, and re-enroll in their program. This is a genius business model, but it doesn't leave the person trying to lose weight with much hope. As a result, people who seek to lose weight often turn to their physician for advice.

I am proud to say that I worked with some of the very best primary care physicians in the country during my time at Massachusetts General Hospital. These brilliant physicians provided truly excellent patient care to those who were sick and were very dedicated to keeping their healthy patients feeling well by preventing the development of chronic disease. However, they, like all physicians, were trained to treat illness by prescribing medications and by providing expert advice to patients. A very small fraction of their time in medical school was spent learning about nutrition and exercise, and there was no time spent learning about how to coach patients to come up with their own weight-loss strategies. In fact, studies show that because of this lack of training, physicians are likely to provide advice to patients based on their personal experience with diet and exercise[1]. For instance, if your physician likes to take a spin class and had success losing weight by eating a low-carb diet, he/she is most likely going to advise you to purchase a Peloton bike and to avoid eating carbs. Therefore, although well-intentioned, your physician, and any "expert" for that matter, is most likely not the best source for weight-loss counseling.

So, if I'm suggesting that you skip the fad diet, avoid the pricey pre-packaged food program, and take your physician's weight loss advice with a grain of salt, how are you supposed to lose weight? The answer is to look within. No, I'm not trying to get all touchy-feely or deep and spiritual but I am trying to express that you need to come up with your own plan in order to say goodbye to the weight you want to lose and to keep it off forever. The common thread that links the trendy diet, the pre-designed meal plan and expert advice are that *someone else* has come up with a one-size-fits-all plan for the masses and is now asking you to follow it religiously, with the expectation that you will figure out how to fit their plan into your life. As you know, this can work for a short period of time if you are willing to wedge someone else's plan into your life. But when it becomes too tough to keep up with, or you just get sick of following someone else's plan, the wheels will fall right off. However, this trap can be avoided by flipping the script on this strategy through self-designing your own weight-loss plan, a plan that you believe in, which fits within the constraints of your life, and is a plan that you can maintain for the foreseeable future.

Your Own Plan is the Best Plan

The year after I graduated with my bachelor's degree I moved home from college, along with everyone else I knew, to live with my parents in order to save money while working at an entry-level job. This migration back to my suburban hometown was, of course, practical, but this change left a lot to be desired when it came to a social life. I had grown accustomed to spending my weekends enjoying the thriving social scene at the University of New Hampshire. Each weekend at UNH brought the opportunity to make new friends and the potential to meet someone I might be interested in dating. However, after breaking up with my college girlfriend and spending the better part of a year seeing the usual familiar faces over and over again, at the same handful of townie bars, my prospects for meeting a love interest were meager at best. But by some miracle, my friends and I went to a bar a few towns over from where we lived and I met a cute, intelligent girl, named Sarah, who had also recently graduated from college and was living at home.

Sarah and I exchanged numbers and eventually, we made plans to meet up for ice-cream. When I arrived at the ice-cream stand to meet Sarah I was teeming with anticipation around the possibility that this date could bring some excitement and, who knows, maybe even a girlfriend, into my newly adopted sleepy suburban life. After greeting each other and ordering, Sarah and I sat down to eat our ice-cream and get to know one another. We shared stories about college and our families and discovered several common interests, which only added to my enthusiasm toward her. Then Sarah told me that she was currently working as a dental hygienist and inquired about my oral care practices by asking "how often do you floss?" I replied, as most twenty-two-year-old males right out of college would, by smiling and saying, "oh, I don't really floss." Boy, was this a mistake. Sarah followed up my reply by proceeding to lecture me on the merits of flossing, and she insisted that I start flossing daily, to the point where she made me agree to start that very night. I politely agreed and when our date ended, she asked if I would call her. I said I would and we parted with a hug.

So, here I am with the opportunity to begin dating an attractive and intelligent woman, with no other prospects in sight for the foreseeable future. Seems like a no-brainer, that I would call her for a second date, right? Wrong. All people, including the twenty-two-year-old version of myself, recoil when they are told what to do. So much so that they would throw away the possibility of dating someone that they otherwise are extremely interested in just to avoid having someone else's ideas forced upon them. This human reaction to revolt against directives that we have yet to assimilate as our own ideas seems to be universal in nature. Since this response is so ingrained in our DNA, it is essential that we keep it in mind when choosing a weight-loss plan. Therefore, in order to achieve your ideal weight and maintain this weight, you must come up with your own weight-loss and maintenance plan, rather than taking someone else's advice or adopting their pre-designed plan. Is this resonating with you? I hope so, but whether it is or isn't hitting home yet, I believe that it is important to explore the behavioral science behind why creating your own weight-loss plan is so important before moving forward. Oh, and just for the record, I did call Sarah to tell her that there wouldn't be a second date (lucky for me since I am now married to the most amazing woman), and I now floss five days a week, but I didn't start flossing until years later when, yes, it was my own idea.

Behavior Change Theory

The methods described in this book combine several behavior change theories into an actionable plan that, if followed, will help you to form sustainable habits. Adopting these sustainable habits will facilitate the loss of significant amounts of weight and the maintenance of this weight loss. The predominant behavior change theories that will be utilized to help you build your own sustainable plan are Choice Theory, The Theory of Planned Behavior, and Goal Setting Theory.

Choice Theory, derived from the work of Dr. William Glasser, is based on the premise that every individual only has the power to control their own choices and no one can control another person's behavior. This theory illustrates why we often revolt against others' suggestions when they try to control our choices. This is exactly what happened when Sarah tried to push me to adopt her suggestion to start flossing. Other examples of this theory in action are when a parent tells their child to clean their room or when an adult child decides that their elderly parent is no longer fit to drive and takes their keys away. Typical outcomes of these attempts to control another person's behavior are that the child ends up having a habitual messy room and that the elderly parent takes the keys to their car in order to hit the road for a defiant joy ride. The bottom line of this theory is that no one likes to be told what to do and that a person will not adopt a sustainable behavior change shift until the decision to make a change becomes their own. Similarly, the Theory of Planned Behavior suggests that people can successfully change their behavior if they believe the change is achievable.

The Theory of Planned Behavior was first proposed by Icek Ajzen in 1985 in his article "From Intentions to Actions: A Theory Of Planned Behavior." The Theory of Planned Behavior is multilayered but for the purposes of this book, we will focus on the piece of the theory that suggests that people are much more likely to attempt to change their behavior when they feel that they can successfully enact the change. In other words, you are much more likely to successfully make a behavior change if you believe that the change is achievable. This theory highlights the importance of designing your own weight-loss plan because if the plan is self-designed it should only be composed of behavior changes that you believe are meaningful and achievable. This theory ties in perfectly with Goal Setting Theory.

In the 1960s, Dr. Edwin A. Locke developed Goal Setting Theory, which established that goals that are difficult to achieve and goals that are specific tend to increase performance more than goals that are not[2]. Later, Locke further developed his theory by identifying three components that lead to goal setting success: self-efficacy, commitment to others, and the perceived importance of the anticipated outcomes if the goals were to be attained[3]. Putting these pieces together, this theory suggests that if the goal you set is important to you, if you believe that you can achieve the goal, and if you incorporate a form of external accountability into your plan, you are much more likely to reach your goal.

While working with my patients at MGH, I used the principles of Choice Theory, the Theory of Planned Behavior, and Goal Setting Theory in combination with proven scientific nutrition and exercise techniques to help people build their own weight-loss plans. By supporting patients to shift their own behavior in a meaningful and sustainable fashion, they were able to lose significant amounts of weight and keep it off. These techniques will be shared with you over the course of this book so that you too will be able to create your own successful and sustainable weight loss plan.

Lose the Weight and Keep It Off

Prior to accepting a position at MGH, I was working as an exercise physiologist at Boston Medical Center's Cardiovascular Center. At Boston Medical Center (BMC) I worked predominantly with patients who had suffered a cardiac event and/or had developed cardiovascular disease. Often the patients who were referred to my care were feeling quite ill, in the process of recovering from cardiac surgery, and/or were traumatized from experiencing a recent heart attack. As their physiologist, it was my job to teach them how to exercise, eat correctly, and lose weight so that they didn't suffer another cardiac event or need a second surgery.

I must say I was quite good at this job. My patients would visit the cardiovascular center several days a week and during these visits, I would dutifully set their treadmill speed for them, tell them how long to exercise for, tell them when to change exercise machines, tell them how much weight to lift, tell them how many reps to lift them for, and I would even hand them the correct weights to lift. I'd also track their weight, review their diet with them, provide education on a heart-healthy diet, and share strategies for weight loss with them. Typically, after twelve to sixteen weeks of this type of care, my patients would graduate from our program having lost weight, having made changes to their diet, and with a much stronger heart, and stronger muscles. At graduation, my patients would often leave my care by departing with words of gratitude, a card that outlined their thanks, and a hug. I'd proudly hang their cards up in my office and leave work feeling satisfied with all that I had done for my patients.

However, after working for several years at BMC I noticed that a lot of my graduates were being re-referred to our program because they had undergone another surgery or suffered a second heart attack. What had gone wrong? I had poured my soul into their care, educated them on everything they needed to know, and developed a holistic plan for them to follow. In retrospect, it is easy to see what went wrong. I did all the work by creating their plan, telling them exactly what to do, monitoring their progress, and making adjustments to their plan. I also took all of the credit for the progress they made. For all of these reasons, the habits that were developed while they were under my watchful eye disintegrated once they left our program only to resume their previous lifestyle habits, which were the same habits that had led them to our program in the first place. After going through this cycle with several of my patients I became certified as a Wellcoaches Health Coach and accepted a position with MGH Primary Care, determined to support my patients in a new and more effective way.

I arrived at MGH in 2011, which was a very exciting time in healthcare. The Affordable Care Act had taken hold and there was a great deal of optimism surrounding a shift in the patient care delivery model. Specifically, primary care providers, including those at MGH, were starting to experiment with the "patient-centered medical home" model, a model that focuses on building relationships with patients in order to provide more comprehensive care. Furthermore, MGH was at the top of its game as an institution and the hospital was looked at as a leader in the development of healthcare delivery models. In fact, during most of the years that I worked at MGH from 2011–2016, it was ranked as the best or the second-best hospital in the country by *U.S. News and World Report*.

During that same time frame, MGH's Ambulatory Practice of the Future, a patient-centered medical home serving MGH employees and their spouses, was consistently ranked as the hospital's top-performing primary care practice. I was, of course, proud to join such a well-respected and innovative practice, and by doing so I became one of the first health coaches integrated into a primary care setting in the country. My primary role within the practice was to support patients in changing their lifestyle habits in order to help them avoid developing cardiovascular disease and diabetes.

Shortly into my tenure at MGH, I realized that although patients were being referred to me for a variety of reasons: high blood pressure, high cholesterol, prediabetes, etc., 95 percent of these patients wanted to focus on weight loss. In response to this need, I set out to develop a method that would allow patients to build their own weight-loss plan in a sustainable fashion so that they could lose the weight they desired and keep it off for good.

After years of working with hundreds of patients seeking to lose weight and through the training I received from Wellcoaches, I was able to determine which components of a weight loss plan are essential in order for people to achieve and sustain significant weight-loss results. These components include:

1. Conducting a self-assessment
2. Identifying one's values

3. Creating an "ideal wellness vision"

4. Identifying where gaps exist among one's values/vision and one's behaviors

5. Creating a plan that includes a vision, S.M.A.R.T. goals, and accountability

The research I conducted while at MGH shows that when you combine these essential behavioral components with evidence-based diet and exercise techniques that have been proven to facilitate weight loss, the results are remarkable.

In the largest study that I conducted, 98 of my patients who built their own weight-loss plan were compared to 123 patients who received weight-loss advice from their primary care physician. The group of patients who built their own weight-loss plan lost an average of 7.24 percent of their initial body weight and the patients who received advice from their doctor on how to lose weight lost less than 1 percent of their initial body weight[4]. In other words, the patients who followed these weight-loss plan guidelines in order to develop their own weight- loss plan lost over 150 percent more weight than those patients who received weight-loss advice from their primary care physician.

These results, which occurred over a twelve-month period, are quite significant on their own, but what brings even more meaning to these results is when you examine these patients' weight two years after they created their own weight loss plan. The weight that these patients lost over the initial twelve-month period was essentially kept completely off as on average only .6 pounds were gained back two years later[4]. In other words, of the ninety-eight patients examined in this study, all of whom followed the techniques outlined in this book, a great deal of them lost in excess of 50 pounds, several losing over 100 pounds, and nearly all of them maintained the weight they had lost. These results are quite contrary to most weight-loss plans/programs which are designed to yield very fast and very short-lived weight-loss results.

As mentioned previously, the main reason nearly every weight-loss program produces very temporary results is that they are prescriptive in nature. As we all now know, nobody likes to be told what to do and it seems to be in our DNA to react to most directives with distaste. For the small minority of people who comply with directives, the results of prescribed weight-loss programs tend to be underwhelming and very short-term, as even these very compliant people do not fully adopt the instructed lifestyle changes like they would if they had come up with the plan themselves. For these reasons this book is going to read very differently from any other weight loss book that you've ever read.

In the chapters to come, you will literally create your own weight-loss plan using the same researched-based behavioral change methods that my patients used at MGH. You will also learn what specific dietary and exercise methods have been proven to promote weight loss so that you can determine which of these methods should be included in your plan. By the end of the book, you will have designed your own personal weight-loss plan. This plan will have been built by you, which will ensure that you have ownership over the changes you intend to make and that you will have the knowledge necessary to revise your plan as you go. This approach will help to ensure that you stay motivated and invested in working toward reaching and maintaining the weight at which you feel your best. As you work on creating your own weight-loss plan you'll be introduced to Katy Cabbage, who was one of my first fifty patients at MGH and the coauthor of this book.

Katy used the behavioral change techniques outlined in this book to lose over 140 pounds and has kept it off for the last eight years. By following Katy's story you'll be able to visualize how the science behind these behavioral change techniques can be applied to real-life situations. You'll also have the benefit of gaining insight into how Katy built her own weight loss plan, a plan which you can reference when building your own plan. Through learning about behavioral change weight-loss techniques and by following Katy's journey, by the time you finish this book you'll have the confidence and knowledge necessary to build your own sustainable weight-loss plan.

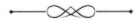

Katy: When I first met Ryan, some of the very first words out of my mouth were, "I don't believe in setting weight-loss goals. So, I won't be making any of those." I was adamant and firm. And he was patient. And I am so grateful he was. Because of the principles he shared with me, and is now sharing with you in this book, he led me on a path of self-discovery that empowered me to have the confidence and vision to see just where my physical, mental, and emotional health could go; including setting and achieving a weight-loss goal. Prior to my meeting him, I had a tendency to get stuck in my thinking and very often fell victim to the belief that there were simply some experiences or health goals that were not achievable for me. He helped me learn just how mistaken I was.

To fully understand where I was mentally when I met Ryan, we have to go back a long way. Back to when I first started putting on weight in childhood. Starting about age seven or so, I started gaining weight faster than my peers. I come from long lines of strong, sturdy folk and my family, to their credit, never made me feel self-conscious about my size. I played sports, I did well in school, I got along well with my peers and had plenty of friends, all the while steadily residing at the top of the weight distribution for my age. As I grew older, because of experiences with peers, I became increasingly self-conscious about my weight and my size. I tried in fits and starts to improve my health (and crossed my fingers it might help me lose weight) many times during my late teenage and early adult years, all to no avail. By the time I graduated college, I weighed 315 pounds and believed that I was destined to be significantly overweight for the rest of my life. I wasn't happy about that prospect, but I had resigned myself to a life of morbid obesity. I truly believed that it was predetermined by genetics, and I could do nothing about it.

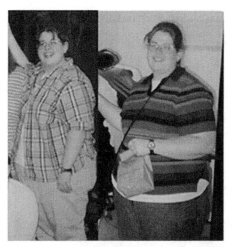

(These pictures show me at my heaviest, circa 315 pounds)

And then, for reasons I still can't quite explain, I made one small change. One spring, after I had started my first real job out of college, I decided to go for a walk every day. It seems small, and it felt small to me at the time, but I had no idea just how much that one decision (and my commitment to that decision) would change the trajectory of my life. I had heard that it takes six weeks for a habit to develop, so I committed to going for a walk every day for six weeks to establish an exercise routine. I had tried to set exercise habits previously: "I'm going to ride five miles on my bike everyday. I'm going to do twenty-five pushups a day for a year. I'm going to do the thirty-day plank challenge." etc. etc. etc. It. Never. Stuck. I'd be enthusiastic for the first few days, but after a time, my resolve fizzled out, and I'd be right back at square one. But, this time something was different. I made my commitment and everyday after I went for a walk, no matter how long it was, I drew a little stick figure on my calendar to record my progress toward my six-week goal. It's important to note that many of those walks could hardly be described as any kind of significant exercise. But I still went. Every day. Sometimes I would annoyedly drive to the walking trail, get out of my car, walk thirty feet down the path, turn myself right around and stubbornly walk back to my car and count that as my "walk." Later we'll discuss how this experience was actually, unbeknownst to me, founded on some scientifically-based principles that helped me sustain this habit.

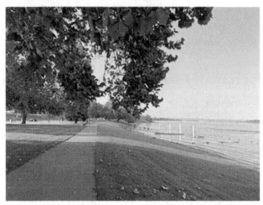

(The walking trail where it all began.)

At the end of six weeks, it was late spring, and I realized that I was actually starting to look forward to my afternoon walks. I began walking a little bit farther each day. Eventually, I discovered there were mile markers on the trail I'd been walking on all these weeks. It was fun to see how far I was walking. I increased my walks to two miles at a time. Then three miles. I started listening to specific podcasts while I was on my walks. I made a rule for myself: I was only allowed to listen to those podcasts if I was walking. Talk about motivation! During this time, I paid little or no attention to my weight. I didn't own a scale and was still convinced that I had no control over my weight. And besides, I knew I was destined to be overweight for the rest of my life.

Over the course of the next few years, my health slowly improved. I still didn't weigh myself, and I certainly wasn't going to the doctor regularly at that time, but I could tell my health was improving because of how I felt. I was able to do things physically I hadn't been able to do for a long time, like comfortably ride a bike or walk four to five miles at a time. My clothes started feeling looser on my body. I continued to ignore my weight. I changed nothing about the way I was eating. After a few years, I moved out of state to continue my education. I was still going for daily walks (I had over 200 weeks of stick figures on my calendar by then. I wasn't about to stop!). At some point, it occurred to me that changing my eating behaviors might be useful. I was very resistant to cutting anything out of my diet because of my experiences trying (and failing) to stick to strict food plans earlier in my life. I decided to try and eat foods that weren't heavily processed and to stick to fresh food and whole grains. I didn't cut out dessert, but I tried to eat less sweets than before. And I finally bought a scale. The first time I weighed myself on it, I was 250 pounds. The last time I had been weighed was at the doctor's office five years earlier, and I was 315 pounds. I couldn't believe it! I now weighed 250 pounds! I was excited! But I was also scared. Although I had lost 65 pounds , I didn't feel like I had any control over it. Yes, I had started walking and yes I had gradually started to adjust my eating behaviors, but I was still convinced that genetics had predetermined my weight, and I didn't have a say in it! I considered it sheer luck that, by the grace of God, maybe because of my walks, I had lost 65 pounds. I was afraid to set a specific goal to lose weight because I wasn't sure I knew or understood how in the world I had managed to lose the weight I'd had. Whenever I had tried to lose weight with a specific plan or system, it never ended well (usually with me, frustrated and disappointed, berating myself and drowning my discouragement in junk food). It made me so fearful to set out to lose weight.

With my new eating practices and my continued walks, I managed to lose another 35 pound . Me! I weighed 215 pounds! And then my schooling got really intense. I was overwhelmed and stressed. I started slipping in my eating habits and falling back into my old ways of eating. By the time I finished my graduate program, my weight had crept back up to 235 pounds. I moved to Boston in the Fall of 2013 to work in a research lab for a few years. I had been living the life of a student for the previous five years while I finished my degree, and I was exhausted physically, emotionally, and mentally. Although I had made several positive changes to my health and weight (which I will talk more about later), I was now stalled at this difficult plateau, and my weight was creeping back up to a place I didn't want to be. To be honest, I was terrified. I was convinced that my prolonged plateau in weight (and now its steady climb up!) was boldly declaring to me just how little control I had over my weight. I was scared to lose the ground I had managed to gain and was sure that I was headed back to my predestined 315 pounds. (Or higher!) I was frustrated and embarrassed.

Because I was in a new city, I needed a new doctor, and I happened to land at Massachusetts General Hospital. At my first visit, the nurse practitioner mentioned they offered free Wellness Coaching as part of their practice. As she explained what a Wellness Coach did, all I could think was, "Yeah, no. I don't need anyone telling me what to do." (the very principle Ryan has been talking about in this chapter – yep! He's right! That is exactly how I felt. I did not want anyone telling me what to do). I knew that I was the expert on my life and my body and was annoyed at the thought of anyone trying to tell me what was best for me or my health. And I was sure that was what a dumb Wellness Coach would do. After the nurse practitioner left the exam room, I rolled my eyes about the whole thing, mentally prepared to ignore the entire suggestion. And then, I paused and thought for just a moment. I knew I had stalled in my health journey. I knew I was starting to panic that my weight was going to keep going up without any stopping. I had been so proud of the changes I had made by adding exercise to my life and adjusting my eating habits. I had been so proud of the effects of these changes on my weight, my health, and what I was able to do physically. Stalling in my progress was a hit to my pride, and part of me felt like working with a Wellness Coach was further admission that I really couldn't manage my health by myself. I had a lot of shame about that and could hear the all-too-familiar voice in my head reminding me that I was destined to stay overweight forever, and there was nothing I could do about it.

Somehow I gathered my courage, and when the nurse practitioner came back into the room, I said that maybe I'd be willing to at least meet with the Wellness Coach, but I wasn't going to make any promises about continuing to meet with him. And that's how I started working with Ryan.

As we continue to move through the principles discussed in this book, I'll share what it was like to be on the receiving end of his coaching and guidance (turns out, I did keep meeting with him!). First and foremost, you need to know that this is not a book that will lay out a cookie-cutter plan, tell you to "eat these three foods and you will lose 100 pounds," or hand you a silver bullet on a platter that will make you thin in thirty days. What it **will** do is provide you the necessary guidance to empower you to identify personalized goals that will be specifically tailored to you and your needs. It will help you develop a personalized plan to help you achieve the vision you develop for your health, your wellness, and yes, even your weight. And you'll hear about the day I finally gathered the courage, and, of my own accord, decided to set a weight-loss goal for myself! I hope that by sharing my perspective and experiences along the way, you'll start to believe what I believe now: that anyone can take charge of their health (and their weight) and change their life trajectory. I don't have any superhuman capacity, and I'm not an anomaly. It doesn't mean it's not hard work. Because it is. But, I am 100 percent confident anyone can learn to make small changes and, over time, change their life in a major way.

Introduction Key Takeaways:

- The excess of information and products related to weight loss can make anyone feel confused and frustrated.

- Taking someone else's weight-loss advice or adopting someone else's weight-loss program is unlikely to yield long-term weight-loss results.

- Behavior change theory suggests that creating your own weight-loss plan is the best way to lose weight and keep it off.

- The research that I conducted at Massachusetts General Hospital shows that adopting the behavior change methods, which will be outlined in this book, leads to significant and sustainable weight loss results.

Phase One: Connect

The connect phase is all about exploring your current behaviors, your personal values, and your desired future state. Through this exploration, you'll come to truly and deeply understand why you want to lose weight and how achieving your ideal weight will enhance your life by promoting your personal values. By the end of phase one, you'll have completed an inventory of your current health behaviors, determined your core personal values, and created your "ideal wellness vision."

The first step in this phase is to reflect on your current behaviors by conducting a self-assessment. This self-assessment will focus on the behaviors that are most relevant to achieving successful and sustainable weight loss.

Chapter 1

Step 1: Conducting a Self-Assessment

Presumably, you're reading this book because you are interested in losing weight, which means that your current lifestyle habits are not supporting your desired weight. Therefore, to lose weight and to keep it off, you'll need to make changes to your lifestyle habits that are sustainable. It seems simple enough, right? Yes, but it can be challenging to decide which of your current lifestyle habits are already going well, and therefore you should maintain, and which habits, if changed, will lead to significant weight loss. In order to help you sort this out, we've created a self-assessment tool, which will allow you to take an inventory of your current lifestyle habits.

When you enroll in a predesigned weight loss program, most often, you will not even go through an intake process; instead, you'll immediately be instructed to start implementing a cookie-cutter plan. If you are working with a weight-loss expert, they might ask you a series of questions in order to better understand your current habits before they design a plan for you to follow. This approach is certainly a step in the right direction, but the expert will rarely, if ever, ask for your opinion on what should be included in your plan.

Contrary to these approaches the self-assessment tool that we have designed will allow you to reflect on your current lifestyle habits and later decide which of these habits you are ready to change. With that approach in mind, I'd encourage you to engage in the self-assessment process as if you were building a "menu" of offerings. Later, when you are building your weight-loss plan, you'll select which habits you desire to change from this menu. In order to build a menu that you'll be satisfied with selecting from when you go to design your plan, you'll need to be brutally honest with yourself.

I have never been a big fan of math; in fact, it was typically my least favorite subject each year of school. So, needless to say, when I had the opportunity to cut corners in order to avoid the drudgery of actually learning math, I'd take it. When I was in middle school, an easy way to cut my math homework in half was to look in the back of the textbook, which displayed the answers to 50 percent of the assigned questions. Without giving it a second thought, I would routinely write down these answers on my paper, whether I actually understood the concept or not, which would buy me at least an extra half hour in my afternoon to play outside. But of course, there was a downside to this shortcut.

By mindlessly writing down the answers to the homework problems, I didn't give myself the opportunity to reflect on whether or not I really understood how to solve the problems on my own. This lack of honest reflection left me unprepared when exam time rolled around. When I referred back to my menu of the knowledge I had acquired, in order to apply it when taking the exam, the offerings were pretty scarce. I don't want you to fall into this same trap, and the best way to avoid feeling like you don't have a satisfactory menu of offerings to choose from when you go to build your weight loss plan is to be as honest with yourself as you can when you are completing the self-assessment.

In addition to honesty, it is imperative that you restrain yourself from taking immediate action after you complete the self-assessment. There is a 99 percent chance this scenario is going to play out, so please pay close attention to this warning. After you complete the self-assessment, you will uncover several current lifestyle habits that you would like to change, and you will feel a strong urge to make these changes immediately. Please, resist this urge! There is no doubt that I appreciate your excitement and willingness to make changes, both of which will be put to good use in time, I promise. However, if you jump the gun and get started on making changes before reading the rest of this book, you are setting yourself up to run into several pitfalls. Most notably, if you make changes without the context of a well-designed plan, they are likely to be enacted in an unsustainable fashion. Secondly, by choosing which habits you are going to change before reading the subsequent chapters, you put yourself in danger of making habit changes that may not deliver the weight-loss results you desire. So please, please, please, resist the urge to start making changes right after you complete the self-assessment.

Keeping my two pleas in mind, which are to be completely honest with yourself and hold off on making any immediate habit changes, please complete the self-assessment by visiting

https://weightlostacademy.com/free-weight-lost-self-assessment/.
Once you have completed the self-assessment, tuck it away someplace safe as you'll need to refer back to your results when you build your weight-loss plan. In the meantime, please check out Katy's self-assessment to understand what her lifestyle habits were like when she started her journey.

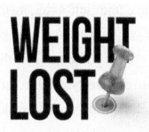

Self-Assessment

DIRECTIONS: This questionnaire contains statements about your way of life, how you've felt, and your habits over the last *3 months*. Please respond to each item as accurately as possible. Indicate the frequency with which you engage in each item by placing an X in one of the following:

Nutrition	Never	Almost never	Once in awhile	Almost always	Always
I eat at least 5 servings of vegetables & fruits daily.			x		
I eat mostly whole grains (brown rice, whole wheat; bread, pasta, and cereals).				x	
I eat low-fat protein (fish, low/non-fat dairy, beans, lean poultry).				x	
I minimize the amount of high-fat foods (full-fat dairy, red meat, baked goods, butter, etc.) in my diet.			x		
I avoid foods high in simple carbohydrates (sugary snacks, junk food, white flour products-rice, bread, pasta, etc.)				x	
I avoid regular drinks with sugar (soda, juice, energy drinks, etc) or diet drinks with artificial sweeteners.					x
I drink at least 8 glasses of water daily.				x	
I eat a high protein breakfast (at least 15 grams) each day			x		
I choose foods that are low in calories but filling (salads, low-fat soups, etc.)			x		
I eat for reasons other than physical hunger (stress, boredom, reward, sadness, etc.)			x		
I eat at least 25 grams (female) and 38 grams (male) of fiber each day			x		
I drink at least one glass (8oz) of water before or during each meal			x		
I eat nutritious meals and/or snacks every 3-4 hours		x			
I eat foods rich in "good", mono and polyunsaturated fats (nuts, eggs, avocados, salmon, olive oil, etc)				x	
I stop eating after I feel full				x	

Exercise	Never	Almost never	Once in awhile	Almost always	Always
I perform cardiovascular exercise at a moderate intensity (brisk walk pace) for at least 150 minutes per week **or** at a vigorous-intensity (jogging pace) for at least 60 minutes per week.				x	
I perform strength training (using weights, tubing, bodyweight) at least 2 days a week.		x			
I prioritize exercise in a way that other responsibilities in my life rarely interfere and cause me to miss a workout				x	
I enjoy exercise					x
I feel that exercise is convenient				x	
I am flexible with my exercise routine (it adapts when my life circumstances change)				x	

Sleep	Never	Almost never	Once in awhile	Almost always	Always
I sleep at least 7.5 hours each night				x	
I maintain a consistent bedtime and wake time				x	
I avoid drinking caffeine after 2pm				x	
I avoid eating high-fat foods before bed			x		
I avoid drinking alcohol before bed				x	
I drink no more than 300-400 mg of caffeine per day (~24 ounces of coffee)					x
I spend time outdoors each day					x

Stress Management and Mental Wellbeing	Never	Almost never	Once in awhile	Almost always	Always
I use strategies (breathing, stretching, relaxation, imagery, meditation) to manage stress daily.			x		
I can release anxiety, worry, and fear without turning to food			x		
I eat due to feelings of boredom, sadness, loneliness, anxiety, or stress			x		
I take time to recognize whether I am eating due to hunger or for other emotional needs			x		
I substitute other behaviors in place of eating when I feel the urge to eat due to my emotions			x		
I experience symptoms of generalized anxiety (feeling nervous, anxious, or on edge, not being able to stop or control worrying)			x		
I experience symptoms of depression (little interest or pleasure in doing things, feeling down, depressed or hopeless)				x	

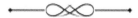

Katy: Before I even met with Ryan for the first time, he emailed me the self-assessment and asked me to fill it out so that we could discuss it when we met at our first appointment. My first thought was "Ugh." I worried that it would simply highlight all the ways I was a slacker and be another source of pain, reminding me of all the ways I was coming up short in regards to my health. I did not like the feeling of being evaluated or judged (who does??) and, before I'd even met him, I assumed that Ryan would be intent on emphasizing all my weaknesses. You may be feeling a bit like that right now. But, I want to remind you that there are likely some things you **are** doing that are contributing positive things to your health. The self-assessment is there to help you identify those things as well as the things you might struggle with. It's designed to help provide you a fuller perspective than perhaps you currently have. Chances are extremely good that you will be pleasantly surprised by things you're already doing that are helping your health. And chances are extremely good that you'll find some areas that you might want to work on.

Back in 2013, when I sat down to complete the self-assessment, I knew I had already established some habits I was proud of. (and I had the stick-figure laden calendar pages to prove it!) I hoped that I would be able to showcase things that were working for me. I am grateful that I was able to fill out the self-assessment in private, ahead of time, on my own. I needed to have the time and the space to fully reflect and consider my behaviors and thoughts without feeling rushed, intimidated, or embarrassed with someone looking over my shoulder while I completed it. You have the opportunity to similarly sit down and personally reflect and conduct your own assessment of your habits, including weaknesses **and** strengths. Try and find a quiet time and space where you can thoughtfully consider your answers to each of the questions. Taking the time to be brutally honest with yourself is key.

The self-assessment is broken down into five main categories: Life Balance and Satisfaction, Physical/Nutrition, Exercise, Weight, and Health Responsibility. As I started perusing the self-assessment when I first received it from Ryan, I was encouraged that the "weight" category seemed to have the smallest emphasis because there were only three questions in that section. Given my history, I was not interested in my weight being a focus of my wellness coaching. At the end of the self-assessment, I said as much when I was asked to respond to an inquiry about what I was most interested in working on. "I am hesitant to set specific weight-loss goals . . . " I was unaware of how much my ideal weight was wrapped up in the other categories.

Completing the self-assessment was an important step. First of all, it helped me realize that while there were some things that I could identify as an area of weakness and/or inexperience, there were definitely other areas where I was feeling like I was doing okay. At that time, there were certain areas of exercise that I had gotten really good at. (I was exercising daily) Still, there were parts of exercise that the self-assessment helped shine a light on for me that I might be missing (stretching regularly? That had never occurred to me!) Although your self-assessment, of course, will look different than mine, I suspect your experience will be similar. Digging deep into multiple health and wellness areas will give you important information about yourself – both in terms of areas that you are feeling okay about and areas that you may decide to start tackling over the next few months.

The self-assessment also served to validate things that I already believed about my health journey, most importantly: True health is about much more than burning more calories than you eat or achieving a certain number on a scale. Health and wellness also needed to take into account things like how I was managing stress in my life (a not-so-strong area for me) and whether or not I was getting enough sleep (which I was doing pretty well at!). It provided insight into healthy habits that I felt confident in (I was exercising quite regularly) and other habits that maybe weren't helping me be where I wanted to be (I almost always watched TV while I ate). I appreciated the process and tried hard to be very honest with myself while I filled out the self-assessment even though it felt rather scary to be so vulnerable. Some of my answers brought a sense of guilt and shame (why did I still struggle with eating foods I KNEW were not good for my health?). But, being open and honest with myself helped lay it all out on the table, and it gave me a place to think about where to start.

Before we move on, one last thing. I echo Ryan's sentiment about resisting the urge to jump in and try to tackle everything at once. I well understand that feeling of seeing where I'm struggling and feeling SO ready to get to where I want to be. It was so important for me to realize that achieving true change in my health and wellness was going to take TIME (and it D.I.D. take time). As human beings, most of us are just not very good at managing a lot of change at one point, myself included. And unfortunately, as human beings, we're VERY good at getting discouraged when we don't master things quickly, myself included. Perhaps you've experienced that before. I have. Once you've completed the self-assessment, take a look over what it teaches you about <u>you</u>. What are you doing well already? What are the areas that are a bit more challenging for you? Is there anything there you're proud of? Is there anything you are excited about working on? Pondering all of these questions is important. It will help remind you there are things to celebrate, and there are also things to work on. And all of that is okay.

What's Next?

Completing the self-assessment process is certainly an essential step towards designing an effective weight-loss plan. Another crucial step is to better understand your personal values. In the next chapter, you will learn about the importance of building a weight-loss plan that supports your personal values, and you will add the values you hold most closely to your plan.

Chapter One Key Takeaways:

- Conducting a self-assessment will allow you to honestly reflect on your habits.

- The result of your self-assessment will be used later in this book to create your weight- loss plan.

Chapter One To-Do List:

✓ Complete your self-assessment

Chapter 2

Step 2: Identify Your Personal Values

Why do you want to lose weight? Take no more than five seconds and answer this question. Okay, now hold onto this answer because I'm going to ask you this question again at the end of this chapter, and I want you to look back to see if your answer has changed.

Answering this simple question in order to express why you want to lose weight might seem like a needless task, especially since you probably wouldn't be reading this book if you weren't interested in losing weight. However, taking the time to deeply and meaningfully answer this question is actually one of the most important, if not the most important, step you will take in your journey toward reaching your ideal weight.

To fully answer this question you will need to discover your "true why." Identifying your true why will require you to press yourself to look beyond your surface-level answer to the question: Why do you want to lose weight? In order to move beyond your initial answer to this question, you'll need to understand how your desire to lose weight is driven by what you value most in life, otherwise known as your personal values.

The term personal values can be interpreted in numerous ways. In this book, we will be defining personal values as: one's judgment of what is important in life. Over the years, the vast majority of my patients were able to reach their ideal weight by applying the techniques that will be laid out for you in the chapters to come. However, several of my patients did not reach their goals. After analyzing this group of patients, a common theme discovered in hindsight was that they did not make a strong connection between their desire to lose weight and their personal values.

Reflecting on these cases individually, there were instances when the patient was unable to share deeply and honestly what they truly valued. There were also times when I failed to ask the right questions in order to push them to dig deep enough, and there were also times when it was a combination of both of these missteps. In any case, in my experience, the individuals who were able to make the connection between their personal values and their weight-loss goals achieved significantly better results when compared to those who were not. These experimental findings are also backed up by theories rooted in the work of positive psychology.

The study area known as positive psychology is defined as "the study of what makes life worth living[5]." What makes life worth living? Or in other words, what are the factors that contribute the most to a well-lived and fulfilling life? The answers to these questions are different for everyone. By answering these questions, you can begin to define your own personal values.

Your personal values define who you are and what is most important to you as a person. These values should establish where you invest your time, energy, and resources; however, this is not always the case and if a discrepancy exists between what you value and how you deploy your resources, it leads to personal unrest and often failed attempts to reach your goals. Speaking of goals, it is important to keep in mind that personal values are different from goals. Goals are an object of a person's ambition, and once the goal is achieved, new goals are often set. However, a personal value doesn't have a beginning and an endpoint but rather lives in the fabric of your life.

The Importance of Defining Your Personal Values

Why is defining your personal values crucial to sustainable weight loss? When you practice behaviors, any type of behaviors, in congruence with your personal values, you will feel a sincere sense of meaning and satisfaction. For example, if one of your personal values is continuous learning, then you would, in turn, feel a sense of satisfaction by practicing behaviors such as taking classes, attending seminars, or reading educational texts. However, if continuous learning doesn't happen to be one of your personal values, attending classes or going to seminars would feel like a burden and a waste of time. This same concept applies when adopting behavior changes in order to lose weight. If your personal values aren't connected to the weight-loss provoking behaviors you are attempting to adopt, then you will abandon them once you have achieved your weight loss goal, if not before.

By integrating behavior changes that are in harmony with your personal values, you will not only be able to achieve your weight-loss goals, but you will be much more likely to sustain these behaviors and, as a result, maintain your desired weight for the foreseeable future. Specifically, through understanding and practicing behaviors that hold true to your personal values, you will improve your rate of success in achieving sustainable weight loss in the following ways:

Decision-making will become much easier: Once you have identified your personal values, making decisions becomes much easier because your values provide guidelines for how decisions should be made. Rather than looking at the pros and cons of each choice (i.e., do I lie in bed for an extra twenty minutes or do I get up and exercise, or do I order the french fries or a baked potato as my side dish?), you can easily identify how each option aligns with your values or doesn't. The best decision for you becomes easily identifiable when you look at them in the context of your personal values.

You'll feel confident about how to spend your time, energy, and resources. I'm sure you've heard the phrase before, "you can have anything, just not everything." The essence of this message is true. The key to having anything you want is knowing how to prioritize your resources. If someone hasn't defined their personal values, they tend to prioritize the things they "should" do or are "expected" to do, which often leaves few resources to dedicate to the things that actually matter to them. When someone is able to articulate their personal values, they can begin investing their time, energy, and resources in the things that are important to them instead of wasting these means on trivial matters. For example, when identifying barriers to achieving their weight-loss goals, many of my past patients often referenced not having enough time to exercise or not having enough money to purchase healthy food. Clearly, these can be real barriers to achieving weight-loss goals; however, once these patients aligned how they spent their time and money with their personal values, they found it easy to work past these barriers.

You'll feel more "like yourself." Once you have identified your personal values and you are ready to take action toward living in harmony with these values, you'll feel more at peace with yourself and the everyday decisions you make. This should bring you a sense of calm and confidence. Katy, who you will hear from later in this chapter, often refers to this as "being in her healthy and happy headspace."

The Danger of Not Defining Your Personal Values

Hopefully, by now, you feel that it is worth your time to define your own personal values before moving forward with creating your weight loss plan. However, let's consider the downside of bypassing this step if you are still on the fence. The three primary dangers that you would be exposing yourself to if you decide not to define your personal values are a loss of motivation, empty goal achievement, and difficulty with weight maintenance.

Let's face it, motivation is the name of the game when it comes to sustainable weight loss. But motivation can be fleeting if it isn't tied to something more meaningful than a number on the scale. If your motivators to lose weight are connected to short-term goals like looking good for an upcoming vacation or to fit into a dress for your friend's wedding, they will lead to short-term results. On the other hand, if your goals are connected to your personal values, which are sewn into the fabric of your being, they will be able to motivate you in order to make sustainable changes. Not only does not connecting your weight-loss goals to your personal values put you at risk for losing motivation, but it can also make goal achievement feel empty.

Early in this chapter, I mentioned that there were several instances in which my patients did not make the connection between their weight-loss goals and their personal values. One of these patients, in particular, sticks out in my mind because of the significant weight she lost in a very short period of time, which was immediately followed by rapid weight gain. I'll never forget Amy standing on the scale in my office, looking blankly, with a slight sense of sadness, at the number on the scale. This number represented the weight that she had always desired to be. When I asked her how she was feeling, she said "empty." Amy went on to tell me that she always thought that seeing that number on the scale would make her happy but in fact, she felt "let down" because the number on the scale didn't make her feel any differently. Looking back, I should have anticipated this lack of joy because although strongly motivated to reach this "magic number," Amy did not take the time to connect how her life would be better, through supporting her personal values, if she reached her goal weight. By skipping this step (and by me letting her skip this step), Amy's weight-loss success added little value to her life and, as a result, made the idea of maintaining this weight meaningless.

Oftentimes the weight-loss process can be exciting, especially if you see the scale tick down on a regular basis, but weight maintenance is a different story. Weight maintenance takes long-term determination and commitment that can only be conjured up when it is truly meaningful for you to maintain this weight. If you have connected your weight-loss goals to your personal values, committing to maintaining your goal weight should not be a problem. However, if you have skipped this step, as Amy did, it becomes nearly impossible to commit to keeping up with the healthy behaviors that lead you to achieve your goal weight. In fact, as I mentioned, Amy didn't see the value in maintaining her goal weight, which in retrospect makes sense because she didn't perceive her life as being better, so she abandoned nearly every behavior change that she had made and gained all of the weight that she had lost back in just a matter of months. As they say, hindsight is 20/20, and in this case, this cliché certainly holds up.

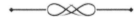

Katy: At the beginning of this book, I explained that when I first met Ryan, I was adamant that I was not interested in setting a weight-loss goal in the form of achieving a particular number on a scale. I want to believe it was because some part of me, although I surely didn't recognize it at the time, was well aware that losing weight for the sheer sake of losing weight was not going to bring me long-lasting happiness. I was convinced I didn't have much control over the number on the scale, so it felt very discouraging to put all my happiness hopes into something I felt I had little control over. Second of all, if I was only invested in my health so long as my weight was going down, then what did it mean if my weight didn't change, or worse – went up!?? Did that mean I should just hang the whole thing and resign myself to a life of dissatisfaction without any joy? Of course not! But it took time to understand how a weight-loss goal fits into the overall picture of my personal values.

Keeping my personal value and worth separate from how much I weighed was very important to me. If I was only going to feel successful in my achievements, if my weight went down, again, what was I going to feel about myself if my weight stayed the same and/or it went up? Or, what did it mean if it temporarily went down to achieve a short-term aim (like losing weight to fit into a dress for a special occasion, say), but then went right back up once the event was over? Did that mean that I was less valuable when my weight went to an undesirable place? Did it mean that my worth was less **until** I lost weight? No. That was untenable to me. By honing in on what I really and truly valued in life – finding my "true why" – I had to dig deep and figure out what it was I wanted to do, who it was I wanted to actually be, and what mattered to me in the greater context of my life. All of which was so much more valuable to me than achieving a number on a scale.

I don't have to tell you that this idea goes counter to what most of society wants you to believe. Every single spring, you can find countless advertisements and internet memes, prompting our yearly obsession with getting ready for the swimsuit season. We all have high school reunions, where we are anxious to prove to our former classmates that we have things together professionally, financially, family-wise, and physically. Maybe we have a family wedding fast approaching, and we are determined to fit into a killer dress. While anyone of these particular events or motivations may actually fit into the framework of your "true why," Ryan helped me look beyond these individual scenarios to the heart of what my **actual** "true why" was. Of course, the journey to figuring out how to articulate this takes time and patience. After you read Ryan's suggestions for how to get there, I'll share what I discovered about my own core values and how they informed my "true why" and helped me achieve what I did not otherwise think possible: losing 150 pounds and keeping it off for eight years (and still going!).

Ryan helped me think a lot about my personal values and how my values were informing the choices I was making (whether positive or negative for my health). I came to him as a pretty independent thinker – I definitely was not looking to him to tell me what to do so that I could do it. But nor had I clearly defined my values in terms of my long-term desires and/or what I wanted to be able to do or be as a result of choices I was making. In truth, it took awhile for me to hone in on what my core values were. It took a lot of pondering, processing, and deciding what was important to me to come to an understanding of what I really wanted or needed in my life. Prior to working with Ryan, I had operated under the framework of goal setting for the sake of achieving those goals. It turns out this was only able to take me so far. Once I started thinking about the core values that were important to me, achieving goals became stepping-stones leading me toward the full depth of the person I wanted to become and the full life I wanted to achieve.

Connecting Your Weight-Loss Goals to Your Personal Values

Connecting your weight-loss goals with your personal values is a three-step process. The first step is to determine your true why or the deeply meaningful reason why you want to lose weight. The second step is to define your personal values, and the final steps are to draw the connection between your true why and your personal values. After completing this process, you will have taken the first step towards building a successful and sustainable weight-loss plan.

Determining Your "True Why."

At this point, if I haven't sold you on the idea of taking the time to define your personal values before you move forward with creating your weight-loss plan, it probably isn't going to happen. However, if you're on board with how important this act is, let's go through the steps you'll need to take in order to clearly and deeply define your own personal values. The first step is to discover your true why.

In order to discover this, you'll need to interview yourself. I'm not talking a light fluff piece interview; this should be a hard-hitting, deeply probing, Mike Wallace-type interview. In other words, I don't want you to accept your first or even second answer as the truth, rather you should keep asking yourself "why" until you unearth why reaching your weight loss goal would mean so much to you. This self-interview will only consist of a maximum of two questions. However, you will have to ask yourself these questions 3-5 times in a row. The two questions that I suggest asking yourself are:

1. Why do you want to lose weight?

2. How will your life be better after achieving your ideal weight?

You can ask yourself one or both of these questions, but chances are you will come up with the same answer to each question. Let's examine what a self-interview may look like by looking back at one of my patient's conversations with himself. When I worked with Bill, he was a 67-year-old man whose goal was to lose 55 pounds. He was referred to me by his primary care physician, who was concerned with his weight gain and his sedentary lifestyle.

Round 1:

Bill: Why do you want to lose weight?

Bill: I want to lose weight so my knees no longer ache.

Round 2:

Bill: Why do you want to lose weight?

Bill: I want my knees to feel better so that I am able to be more active.

Round 3:

Bill: Why do you want to lose weight?

Bill: I want my knees to feel better so that I am able to ride my bike and run around with my grandchildren.

Round 4:

Bill: Why do you want to lose weight?

Bill: I love spending time with my grandchildren, and my weight is prohibiting me from doing this.

Round 5:

Bill: Why do you want to lose weight?

Bill: Spending more time with my grandchildren would make me happy, and achieving losing weight would allow me to do this.

So what do you think, was Bill able to discover his true why during his self-interview? I think he was! He started off with connecting his desire to lose weight to reducing his knee pain, however after several rounds of questioning, he was able to unearth the true reason behind his goal of losing 55 pounds, which was to be able to spend more time with his grandchildren because this would make him happier. Now let's turn our attention to how Bill went about defining his personal values.

Before moving to the next section, please "interview" yourself in order to define your true why for losing weight. Once you have defined your true why please add it to your planning template, which you can download at https://weightlostacademy.com/weight-lost-planning-template/

Defining Your Personal Values

Your personal values are just what they sound like; they are what you personally value most in life. Chances are you haven't given much time, if any, to formally state or write down these values. We all have them, but rarely have we given much thought to what they are, let alone ranked them by importance, which is exactly what I am going to ask you to do now by following this four-step process.

Step 1. Review the following list of values and pick out the ones that you would consider to be on your own personal value list and write them down:

Achievement	Creativity	Excitement	Friendships
Belonging	Learning	Expertise	Growth
Community	Efficiency	Exploration	Hard Work
Compassion	Enjoyment	Family Oriented	Health
Independence	Leadership	Making a difference	Helping others
Service	Simplicity	Spontaneity	Stability
Strength	Success	Teamwork	Uniqueness

Step 2. Add any of your additional personal values that weren't represented in the list offered in Step 1.

Step 3. Now that you have an exhaustive list, please ask yourself the following question: "Will I still consider all of these as my personal values twenty-five years from now?" Then cross off those values that don't meet this criterion.

Step 4. Rank your values in order, starting with the most important at the top. Your top three to five values are considered your "core personal values." Please add these values to your plan template.

After following this same process, Bill's list looked like this:

Bill's Personal Values

1. *Family Oriented*

2. *Leadership*

3. *Health*

Connecting Your" True Why" and Your Personal Values

Now that you have defined your true why and your personal values, it is time to determine how they are connected. Understanding how your desire to lose weight and your personal values are connected will help you create a weight-loss plan, which, once achieved, will bring great joy and meaning to your life. You will also be able to reflect on this connection as a way to motivate yourself to continue working towards your ideal weight when times get tough.

In order to help you make the connection between your true why and your personal values, let's look at Bill's connection. After conducting his self-interview, Bill discovered that his true why was that he wanted to lose weight in order to spend more time with his grandchildren. Additionally, by following the same four-step process that you just went through, Bill determined that his personal values were: being family-oriented, leadership, and health.

So how is Bill's true why connected with his personal values? Well, as Bill explained to me, the things that he values the most in life and that bring him the most happiness are spending time with his family, providing strong leadership, and staying in good health. By reaching his ideal weight, he would be able to spend more meaningful time with his grandchildren. Bill had several grandchildren under ten years old who were always riding their bikes, playing soccer, and playing other yard games whenever they came to visit or when Bill went to visit them. Sadly, during their time together, Bill was forced to stay on the sideline due to his knee pain and low aerobic capacity. However, if he were able to achieve his ideal weight, he would be able to play with his grandchildren. By being physically active with them, Bill would also feel as though he was providing strong leadership by modeling the importance of maintaining an active lifestyle as an older adult. Finally, one of Bill's personal values is to maintain good health. By reaching his ideal weight, Bill would be upholding this value by improving his overall well-being.

As it turns out, Bill's desire to lose weight was very connected to his personal values. I'm proud to share on Bill's behalf that Bill eventually reached his ideal weight, but it wasn't without conflict. There were times, like when his wife got sick, that he took a few steps back; however, Bill was always able to remind himself of why it was so important for him to reach his ideal weight by reflecting on the connection between his weight-loss goal and his personal values.

So, how is your why behind the why connected to your personal values? Take time to give this question some thought and talk it out with someone you trust if you think this would help. Once you've landed on the answer to this question, please add it to your plan template. You, too, can have your own "Bill like" story by creating a weight-loss plan built on a foundation connected to your personal values.

Do you remember the question I asked you at the beginning of this chapter? It was: why do you want to lose weight? Has your answer evolved? I trust that it has.

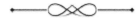

Katy: As you complete this exercise of finding your "true why" and connecting that to your personal values, please be aware that you will likely need to revisit this exercise several times as you progress in your own journey. That's the way it was for me. As I mentioned earlier, it took me time and experience to hone in on exactly what it was that was important to me. This was a difficult process for me. First of all, I had to remind myself that I was seeking to figure out MY "true why," not anybody else's. I am a people-pleaser by nature. I am quick to defer my needs/wants to others around me if I think it will make them happy, more content, and/or more at ease. The process of finding **my** True Why required me to disregard what anyone else thought I should do, who they thought I should be, and where they thought I should be going. This included Ryan. In retrospect, it was so important for me to take ownership of what I needed to do to benefit my own health. If the only reason I am making particular health choices is because a doctor/health coach/friend/social media influencer says I should, I am not taking responsibility for my choices. I'm allowing someone else to decide what is best for my life. Let's be honest; at first, it's far more comfortable to abdicate that responsibility to someone else. It's kind of nice to have someone tell you what to do. It's hard work to make big life decisions like this; it's overwhelming to have to generate ideas about what will bring happiness and fulfillment to your life; it's seemingly easier to let someone else dictate a plan that you just follow. It can feel more comfortable initially to let someone else make these decisions but, I believe doing so inevitably leads to one of two outcomes: 1) resentment over someone else controlling your life, or 2) laying the blame on another party when you don't achieve the outcome. In both cases, you're left feeling powerless and frustrated. Taking responsibility for identifying what **my** core values are has been **so** empowering. I have learned that, if there's something I really want to achieve/become/experience, I am the only one that can reliably make that happen. It becomes my "true why."

Finding my "true why" forced me to ask myself deep and personal questions that required a lot of self-reflection and soul-searching. Some questions that I asked myself:

1. What are things or experiences I'm really hopeful can happen for me?

2. Are there certain accomplishments I long to achieve?

3. Are there painful experiences from my past that are making me afraid to try things now?

4. Are there people I'm trying to impress? Trying to avoid disappointing?

5. Am I afraid of disappointing myself?

6. What are the things that would make me proud? Confident?

In the end, often I wasn't able to get to the core value/true why right away. It took me several iterations to figure out the things that were truly important to me and which things I was willing to dismiss. Over time, I came to three core values that, even today, inform almost every health decision I make.

1. I highly value being able to share experiences with family and friends.

2. I want to live a life without fear.

3. My health choices need to be sustainable and practical.

The first core value I identified centered around how important it was for me to be able to participate and share experiences with family and friends. In essence, I wanted to be able to confidently accept invitations to participate in activities, events, and experiences with those I love without having to decline because of any physical limitations. In essence, I didn't want to opt-out of really living because I couldn't physically participate in these things. How did I identify this as a core value? It really came about as the result of a lot of reflecting back on my life. To fully understand this, we need to take a little trip back in time to my teenage years.

Prior to adolescence, I was an active kid: I played sports, I swam all the time, I rode my bike all over the neighborhood and loved it. Sometime in late middle school and early high school, I started to become rather self-conscious about my physical capabilities and my physical appearance. With little conscious awareness, I began self-selecting out of situations that might put me in a position where I felt self-conscious about my physical capabilities or my physical appearance. And thus became my status quo for the next several years of my life. I turned down invitations to swimming parties, school dances, and playing on intramural sports teams, even just for fun. I strategically made sure I "had plans" when friends were planning outdoor adventures to go hiking, kayaking, or to the lake. I conveniently "forgot" my bathing suit when friends were getting together at someone's house who had a pool. I even began to convince myself I didn't actually like doing any of these things. That couldn't have been farther from the actual truth.

As I began to lose weight and gain strength physically in my twenties, I was still hesitant to accept invitations to participate in physical activities because I was sure I would not be able to keep up and/or actually do the activity. I will forever be grateful to kind and trusted friends who encouraged me to start participating, **really** participating, in life again in my mid-twenties. One friend was particularly pivotal. She invited me to go kayaking, and without giving it any thought at all, I turned her down. She pressed the issue and asked me why I didn't want to go. I told her, "Because there's no way I can kayak. I've never done it. I don't think I'm strong enough to paddle myself around the water. I'll probably get swept downstream. And besides, heaven knows I won't be able to fit in that little seat hole in the kayak!" She didn't tease me. She didn't discredit my concerns. All she said was, "Katy, I know you can do this." Oh, how grateful I am for her encouragement! I checked with her, "Do you honestly think I can kayak?" I didn't want her to patronize me and give me baseless encouragement. I needed her honest assessment. She nodded in the affirmative. She actually believed I could do it. And, for the first time in several years, I voluntarily tried a brand new physical activity with no sure knowledge I would be successful. So, I went kayaking. And I LOVED it. I loved getting to experience something I'd only seen other people do (but it had sure looked fun!).

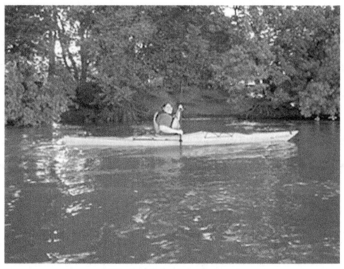

(My first kayaking adventure.)

Thus began my love for adventuring in so many forms: hiking, cycling, backpacking, swimming in the ocean, traveling, etc. I have since come to realize one of the core values that keeps me choosing health is so that I can participate in physical experiences and activities with people that I love. It enriches my life in so many ways, and I try to say "YES!" whenever I can to these invitations.

Another core value I've identified is wanting to live without fear of limitations from my body. I have spent a good chunk of my life fearing situations where my body's sheer size prevented me from fully participating in life. The day that I had to get off a rollercoaster because my body prevented the lap bar from clicking into place was mortifyingly unpleasant. In my teenage years, I started to become wary about seating situations that might be too narrow, too tight, or simply unfeasible. I tried to squish myself as far away from my seatmate on the bus or the airplane, so less of my body would brush against their body. I remember one particularly harrowing night when I couldn't get myself out of the back seat of my friend's two-door car. I heaved and huffed and angled and stretched every way I could think of and still, after ten minutes, was stuck in the back of that dang car. If it seems funny to you now, I assure you there was nothing funny about it in the moment. I knew I had gotten myself INTO that car, why in the world could I not get out of it? In sheer desperation and fear that they'd have to call the fire department and use the jaws of life to get me out, in one last herculean effort I managed to extricate myself from the car. I made a mental note to **never,** under any circumstances, get into the back seat of a two-door car again. I hated being afraid of situations I might get myself into. The most unnerving were the situations I couldn't anticipate (like getting stuck in the backseat of a car? Who does that??). Again, I started opting out of participating in life.

But, as I started to experience the benefits of a body that was simply smaller in size, I realized that I was no longer fearing situations and I really liked that! The thought of living a life without fear of being too large, being too slow, and/or being physically unable to achieve something was definitely a life I wanted to live. And, now I'm here!

The last core value that I identified that was really important to me was ensuring that any changes I was making were things that I felt were good for my health. For me, that meant that these changes were sustainable and practical in my life. I was not willing to incorporate any health decisions/behaviors that were related to fad-diets, fad-workouts, etc., because I knew they would not likely be sustainable. As I was on my health journey, there were countless people who had advice and suggestions for how I could continue my journey of health. Many of these came from well-meaning and kind friends and loved ones who, I believe, honestly had my best interest in mind. But, the more I learned on my health journey, the more I was convinced that this was my health journey, and no one else's. I evaluated all kinds of suggestions: eating plans, workout regiments, supplements, etc. I learned to trust my body and my mind and if something didn't feel like it jived with my goals and/or I didn't think it was going to fit into my lifestyle, it was okay to let it go.

Throughout my time working with Ryan, there have been several aha! moments that have helped clarify my core values and my true why. He pointed out to me at some point that I was happiest and most content when my behaviors were consistent with my values, regardless of what was happening on the scale with my weight or otherwise. This is still true. When my behaviors are consistent with the things that I value, I am happy and content. As Ryan mentioned, I call this "being in my happy and healthy headspace."

Here is what I have learned. When I am in a happy and healthy headspace (i.e., when I'm living my "true why"), I have found that several things happen without much effort:

1. I am confident.

2. I am proud of the decisions I am making.

3. I am excited about setting goals.

4. I am hopeful about my future.

5. I feel like nothing is too difficult to achieve.

By contrast, when I am not in this space (i.e., when I am not living true to my core values), I tend to feel the opposite and am more likely to feel:

1. Discouraged by my failings.

2. Overwhelmed by the challenge of choosing health and overwhelmed with life in general.

3. Frustrated with my decisions.

4. Down on my ability to accomplish the goals I've set.

5. Worried about my health future.

Finding your "true why" will take careful reflection and soul-searching. The important thing is to figure out what it is **you** want. No one else can determine that for you. Where do your values lie in terms of your relationships? Your goals? Your health? As you sort out your "true why" you'll hone in on the things that you value the most and, as a result, your life will be enriched in ways that are meaningful and unique to **you**.

What's Next?

In the next chapter, you will go through the process of creating your "ideal wellness vision," which will be built in alignment with your personal values. By creating this vision, you will be painting the picture of your future self, which is genuinely an inspiring process!

Chapter Two Key Takeaways:

- Your personal values define who you are and what is most important to you in life.

- Connecting your weight-loss goals to your personal values will make you more likely to achieve and sustain your desired weight.

- Connecting your personal values to your weight-loss goal will help you stay motivated, will bring deep meaning to the achievement of your goal, and will make it easier for you to maintain your ideal weight.

Chapter Two To-Do List:

- ✓ Define your "true why"

- ✓ Define your personal values
- ✓ Connect your "true why" and your personal values

Chapter 3

Step 3: Create Your Ideal Wellness Vision

In a minute, I will ask you to please close your eyes for twenty seconds and imagine that you are walking on the beach. While you are imagining this stroll on the sand, I want you to consider what you see, what you hear, what you smell, and what you feel. Okay, now please close your eyes, and imagine yourself walking on the beach for the next twenty seconds.

During this exercise, there were areas of your brain that were unable to distinguish if you were actually walking on the beach or just visualizing it. If only taking a beach vacation was this easy! Although you might not be completely feeling refreshed from your twenty-second visualization, the results of numerous studies indicate that whether you imagine an action or you are actually performing it, the areas of the brain involved are very similar.

In this chapter, you will learn about how visualization works, how you can use visualization to help you achieve your weight-loss goals, and you'll create your "ideal wellness vision."

How Visualization Works

Researchers have discovered that when you imagine yourself performing an action, it is your premotor cortex that is most active. For example, scientists measured how physical training and training by visualization affected the strength of finger muscles. Physical training increased finger muscle strength by 30 percent, and visualization alone increased finger muscle strength by 22 percent. Since the subjects did not make any muscle contractions during their visualization training, the change in strength did not come from enhancements in the connection between the brain and the finger muscles, sometimes referred to as "muscle memory," but actually came from the activation of circuits in the central motor system[1].

In a similar study, Brian Clark at Ohio University showed that using visualization has the potential to make your muscles stronger. His study consisted of twenty-nine subjects whose wrists were wrapped in surgical casts for four weeks. During these four weeks, 50 percent of the participants thought about exercising their immobilized wrists, five days a week, for eleven minutes at a time. These participants simply sat completely still and focused their mental energy on imagining that they were flexing their muscles. When the casts were removed, the participants who did mental exercises had wrist muscles that were two times stronger than those who had done nothing at all[2]. Great, you are thinking, you just have to imagine yourself working out and eating better, and you'll lose weight. Well, no, it isn't going to be that easy. But by imagining your ideal wellness vision, what you and your life will look like one year from now, you will be setting yourself up for future success.

At this point, you might be thinking, how does visualization possibly produce these types of results? Well, according to research, visualization, a technique for creating a mental image of a future event, works because neurons in our brains transmit information and interpret imagery as equal to a real-life act. When you visualize an action, your brain transmits an impulse that tells you neurons to conduct the movement. This creates a new neural pathway, which are clusters of cells in our brain that work together to create memories or learned behaviors. The creation of this neural pathway is what gets our body ready to act in a way that is consistent with what we envisioned. This all takes place without having to actually perform the physical act, yet it achieves a very similar result.

For example, suppose your goal is to run your first marathon. In that case, you could use visualization to envision the details of the race before it takes place by imagining yourself starting the race, hearing the roar of the crowd, feeling your sneakers pounding on the pavement as you run, feeling the sun on your shoulders, feeling your breath increase as you push up the final hill, and feeling the sense of pride and excitement as you cross the finish line a minute under your goal time. What does it feel like to pass under the finish banner? Who is there to greet you as you finish? Your family? Friends? Other runners? Imagine the excitement, satisfaction, and pride you will experience after you finish. By imagining yourself in this future reality, you are priming your brain and your body to take the necessary steps that will lead you to this image of your future self.

However, visualization is a double-edged sword as it can also lead to failures if you are visualizing yourself falling short of your goals. As a lifelong Boston Red Sox fan, I can recall numerous epic failures; however, the most famous of all their heartbreaks is when Bill Buckner, Red Sox first baseman, let a ground ball go through his legs during game six of the 1986 World Series, which resulted in a Red Sox loss. The Sox went on to lose game seven and surrender the Series to the New York Mets. Most baseball fans (over a certain age) are aware of this history; however, what very few know is that Bill Buckner envisioned this failure as his future reality.

On October 6, 1986, Buckner was interviewed by WBZ-TV's Don Shane about the pressures of postseason play and said, "The dreams are that you're gonna have a great series and win. The nightmares are that you're gonna let the winning run score on a ground ball through your legs. Those things happen, you know. I think a lot of it is just fate." Now, I have no idea if Bill Buckner spent any time envisioning the ball going through his legs and letting the winning run score but based on his comments, I would guess that he did, especially since that's exactly what ended up happening.

Shifting our focus back to using visualization to foreshadow positive outcomes, I want you to consider how important it is for you to visualize your *desired* future state before creating a weight-loss plan. It's been found that visualization can increase confidence, and self-efficacy, enhance motivation, and prime your brain for success. Before you can believe in a goal, you must first imagine what it looks and feels like to achieve it. You might have heard the saying: "you must see it before you can believe it." Well, this is exactly the case here. When you visualize your desired outcome, you begin to "see" the possibility of achieving it. Through visualization, you can see what life looks like as your "ideal self."

Creating Your "Ideal Wellness Vision"

Now that you understand why visualization is effective and how it works, it's time for you to create your own ideal wellness vision. In order to do so, I would recommend that you follow this four-step process: set a one-year weight-loss goal, envision your ideal self, draft your wellness vision, and review, revise, and compose your vision.

Step 1: Set a One-Year Weight-Loss Goal

For your first visualization, I want you to close your eyes and imagine yourself one year from today, having lost weight. What do you look like? How does it feel to see yourself this way?

Okay, now I'd like you to make this image a little more concrete by infusing some measurables. You can do this by imagining yourself at a future desired weight by asking yourself these questions:

- When you envision yourself stepping on the scale, what number do you see?
- Does this number thrill you?

If not, take an imaginary step off the scale and think of a number that would make you throw your hands up and scream with excitement if you saw it. Okay, now take an imaginary step back on the scale. What number do you see now? Add this number to your planning template because you will need it later.

Step 2: Envisioning Your "Ideal Self"

When you close your eyes next, I want you to return to the image of yourself one year from now, having reached your ideal weight. In order to add the necessary details to this vision, you'll need to paint a picture of your ideal self by writing down the answers to these questions:

- *Appearance*
    - How do you look?
    - How do you feel at your new weight?
    - How do your clothes fit?
    - What size clothes are you wearing?
    - What type of clothes are you wearing?
    - Are there clothes you are wearing that you didn't feel confident in wearing before?
    - How do you feel in these clothes?

- *Activity*
    - What can you do now that you couldn't do at your previous weight?
    - Who are you spending your time with? Has this changed?

- *Values*

- How has this weight loss allowed you to better live by your personal values?

- How has your life been enhanced by reaching this goal?

Step 3: Draft Your Wellness Vision

In order to draft your wellness vision, you are going to use your results from Steps 1 and 2. What makes up your ideal wellness vision is up to you, with the exception of four requirements. The first is that it includes a weight-loss goal. The second is that it should only consist of changes that solely rely on your efforts. What I mean by this is don't create a vision that relies on someone else changing. For example, do not include details like "my husband and I are exercising each day together" or "my wife appreciates how I look in a suit." The third requirement is that your vision reflects your personal values. Finally, the fourth and the most important requirement is that your ideal wellness vision, once reached, should make you feel ecstatic!

Before you begin writing, I'd like you to review Bill and Katy's ideal wellness vision. Here is Bill's vision:

> One year from now, I have lost 55 pounds and weigh 180 pounds. I am wearing size thirty-four pants, a large T-shirt, and my leather jacket that my wife gave me for my fiftieth birthday. I play soccer, go bike riding, and run around with my grandchildren every time that we are together and can do so free from knee pain. I set a healthy example for my grandchildren by exercising on a regular basis.

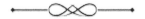

Katy: I'm going to be straight with you here. Creating a wellness vision was one of the most difficult parts of this whole process for me. Why? Before I met with Ryan, I didn't spend a lot of time thinking about my health in a long-term way. I didn't look more than a few weeks out (certainly, never a year!), and I never really envisioned the health outcome if I achieved the goals I set. I knew that I wanted to be thinner at some point. Still, I couldn't figure out what tangible changes I would experience due to being thinner, nor could I figure out what goals would get me there (remember, I didn't feel like I had any control over actually losing weight). It seemed so overwhelming because nothing happened quickly. As a result, the goals I was setting were quite mechanical, rather short-term, and unrelated to any specific health outcome. For example, the first goal I ever set in relation to my health was to go for a walk every day for six weeks. The outcome I looked forward to was not, as one might think, how my body would feel after going for a walk every day for six weeks or even being able to walk a certain distance. The outcome I cared about was being able to look at my calendar filled with the stick figures I drew each day I went for a walk. This is an outcome that literally had nothing to do with how my health or wellness changed over the course of those six weeks. This may seem trivial, but I don't think it is. At this point in time, the outcomes I was looking for were completely detached from any measures of health and wellness. I wasn't connecting the behaviors I was changing with any measurable outcome in how it would impact my life in terms of any kind of long-term vision for myself. Because of this, it was difficult to make long-term sustainable change.

The other factor that made creating a vision so challenging was my resistance to set a weight-loss goal (which, as Ryan points out, is an important part of the vision). In fact, for a whole year, I didn't set a weight-loss goal at all. My vision during that time only included health behaviors that were unrelated to what might happen with my weight. Let's take a look at what my initial vision was for myself:

"Katy is able to perform ten reps of a hanging leg lift. She jogs for three miles without stopping. She plans her meals in advance, and they consist of the right balance of macronutrients."

Please note that this format doesn't exactly follow the plan Ryan laid out above. As a result, my initial success was limited. All the elements of that first vision referred to specific skills I thought I wanted to achieve but really didn't connect with how achieving these things would improve my life physically, mentally, or how they would contribute to my overall wellness. I share this to demonstrate that creating a vision was a process for me and it will very likely be a process for you too. Even though I initially missed the mark, there are some important things about this vision that shed some light about myself. Everything I included was completely under my control. I didn't feel like I could control how much weight I lost but I **did** know I could control whether I could work myself up to being able to jog for three miles.

One of my challenges around envisioning a weight-loss goal was that **I didn't actually know** what my body would look like, feel like, or be like at a lower weight. I had been overweight since the time I was nine or ten-years-old and had been considered morbidly obese since my early teenage years. When I finally decided on a goal weight for my vision, my goal was to weigh less than 200 pounds. It seemed like a satisfying number to finally be in the 100s. When I declared the goal, Ryan asked me to visualize what being 199 pounds would look like in terms of my appearance, what activities I'd be able to do, and how I would feel about myself. I had no idea. It occurred to me that the last time I had weighed 199 pounds was approximately ninth grade. And now I was in my mid-thirties. The only vision I had of a 199-pound version of me was an awkward teenager who was far and away the largest girl in gym class coming in last at every activity. I literally had no idea what 199-pound adult Katy would be like. That made it difficult to amass a vision for myself, because I just couldn't picture her!

But, with Ryan's encouragement and, let's be honest, the use of my imagination, I began thinking through what it was I thought I would be able to do, feel, and achieve in a year-long wellness vision that included weighing less than 200 pounds. Over time, I gained the courage to modify my vision, and I learned to connect my goals with how I wanted to feel physically, mentally, and emotionally and with what I wanted to be able to accomplish. And I ultimately arrived at the following vision for myself, addressing different aspects of my life:

"My weight will be below 200 pounds. I will be able to run a 10K and will be completing strength training three times/week. I will be able to buy new clothes in the regular women's section of the store, instead of the plus-size women's section. I will feel more confident in social situations with friends, coworkers, and dating relationships."

Over the next several years, I continued to adapt my vision of wellness and have expanded it to include things like:

"My weight will be in the 170s and I will regularly hike with friends and family."

"I will accept invitations to do physical activities without hesitation."

"I will wear a bathing suit without fear or shame."

"I will seek out opportunities for dating and social interactions."

Your vision will likely look very different than mine and will require you to reflect and consider the aspects of your health that you want to address to help get you where you want to be. As you take time to reflect, you will likely come to your own epiphanies about yourself that, when faced, will ultimately give you a strong vision of where you want to be one year from now.

Now that you have a sense of what Bill and Katy's visions looked like, please compose your own wellness vision, as you see yourself one year from today.

Step 4: Review, Revise, and Compose Your Vision

Now that you have a working draft, your next step is to review what you have, make revisions, and compose your wellness vision. In order to verify if your vision draft meets the criteria I mentioned in Step 3, you'll need to ask yourself these very important questions:

- Does your vision include a weight-loss goal?

- Does this vision excite me beyond belief? If your answer is no, dream bigger, and make sure to include elements in your vision that would make you feel over the moon.

- Does your vision reflect your personal values? As you are well aware, your weight-loss plan must reflect your personal values in order for you to execute it with success. Additionally, if reaching your ideal wellness vision does not enhance and promote your personal values then why is it worth working toward? In order to ensure that your life will be meaningfully enhanced by achieving your ideal wellness vision, make sure that it is closely tied to your personal values.

- Does achieving your vision only rely on yourself to change? You have the power to make any in your life that you want. However, you cannot change the thoughts or actions of others. Remember, no one wants to be told what to do? To make sure that your wellness vision is 100% within your control, revise any details that count on others altering their beliefs or actions.

Now that you have reviewed and revised your ideal wellness vision, it is time to compose a final product. To do so, please add your ideal wellness to your weight-loss plan template.

What's Next

The ideal wellness vision that you just created will be used as the compass to inform your decision-making during the rest of the creation and execution of your weight-loss plan. Specifically, you will use your wellness vision to guide your path when setting S.M.A.R.T. goals, all of which will be in service to reach this vision. However, before you start setting goals, you'll need to learn more about the behavior changes that have been proven to lead to sustainable weight loss, which is the focus of Phase Two. But before moving ahead, please review the Phase One checklist to ensure that you are ready to move forward.

Chapter Three Key Takeaways:

- Visualization is a technique for creating a mental image of a future event.

- Performing visualization causes our brains to transmit information and interpret imagery as if the act was happening in real life.

- It's been found that visualization can increase confidence and self-efficacy, enhance motivation, and prime your brain for success.

- Creating an "ideal wellness vision" of where you imagine yourself to be one year from now can increase the likelihood of you achieving this desired state.

Chapter Three To-Do List:

- ✓ Set a one-year weight-loss goal.

✓ Draft an "ideal wellness vision."

✓ Review, revise, and compose your vision.

Phase Two: Explore

"There is so much information out there about what you should do to lose weight. How do I know what will actually work"?

This is a question I hear all the time from people who want to lose weight but who are overwhelmed by the amount and often contradictory information they are receiving. Frustrated patients would routinely express things like, "I read that eating eggs for breakfast would help me lose weight, so I started to eat two each morning. But then I heard that eggs are high in fat and could cause weight gain, so I stopped." This is just one example of hundreds that leave people feeling confused and discouraged about trying to do the right things in order to lose weight. This is why, in the Explore Phase, you are going to read about only the most well-researched behavior changes that have been shown to produce weight loss.

You'll start this phase by gaining an understanding of the physiology behind achieving satiety and the best ways to feel full while still reducing your caloric intake. From there, you'll gain insights into emotional eating and how to manage it, and you'll finish the section by learning about how cardiovascular exercise and strength training can help you lose weight. By the end of the Explore Phase, you'll fully understand the behavior changes that, if implemented, will support significant and sustainable weight loss.

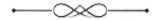

Katy: As someone who spent the better part of my adolescence and early adulthood significantly overweight, I am no stranger to the myriad recommendations that come from friends, family, social media, and society at large for ways one can lose weight and become the picture of health. The constant onslaught of information can be overwhelming and difficult to parse through. Well-meaning friends and associates were often eager to share the diets/workout regimes/lifestyles that led them to lose weight and/or get them in shape for swimsuit season. Perhaps you have experienced that too. As Ryan pointed out, sometimes, these suggestions are in direct contradiction with each other. I often felt overwhelmed by how in the world to figure out who or what was right in this process. I thoroughly appreciated Ryan's approach to this conundrum: He provided me with the scientific basis of how to be physically and psychologically well, which would, in turn, allow my body's physiology to work as it should. Then it was up to me to determine what to implement (and how to implement it) effectively in my own lifestyle.

Chapter 4

Caloric Deficit

My wife and I like to keep our financial planning simple. We always have enough money in our checking account to pay for our normal monthly expenses, mortgage, gas, food, etc., and after those bills are paid, the money we have leftover each month is transferred to our savings account. This savings account grows until we dip into it for extraordinary purchases like furniture, vacations, or home improvement projects. Much like our financial system, your body likes to keep its energy usage straightforward.

Your body prefers to meet all its energy (caloric) needs through daily food consumption. Remarkably, most of the time, you will eat very close to the exact number of calories your body needs to fuel itself over the course of a day. However, when you consume more calories than your body needs, your body will store those calories as fat cells. In the case of my finances, diverting extra funds to my savings account is a good thing, as it causes the balance to increase. But when it comes to energy storage, repeatedly eating more calories than your body expends will cause a buildup of fat stores, which results in weight gain. While on the other hand, the creation of a repeated caloric deficit will result in weight loss.

Much like the process of weight gain, when you boil down the mechanism of weight loss, it is reduced to a pretty simple series of biological events. When you consume fewer calories than your body needs to fuel itself, it will result in the creation of a caloric deficit, which causes your body to break down fat stores in order to meet its energy demands. When this process occurs over and over again, fat stores are routinely broken down in order to be used as energy, which results in weight loss. Pretty simple, right? In some ways, it is; however, we all know that achieving long-term weight loss isn't simple or easy. Later in this book, we will share with you proven behavior changes that, if made, will allow you to create a daily caloric deficit. But let's not get ahead of ourselves; in this section, we will focus on explaining what it means to achieve a caloric deficit and how it promotes long-term weight loss.

How Creating a Caloric Deficit Leads to Weight Loss

By definition, creating a caloric deficit means consuming less energy (calories) than your body needs. But eating five calories less than your body needs each day isn't going to lead to weight loss. However, we do know that there are certain caloric thresholds you must stay under each week in order to lose weight.

In truth, the calorie deficit that you need to maintain in order to lose weight varies from person to person. But thanks to the work of Dr. Max Wishnofsky, we know that as a general rule of thumb, you must create a caloric deficit of at least 500 calories per day in order to lose one pound per week.

Why 500 calories a day, you ask? Well, Dr.Wishnofsky discovered that there are 3,500 calories in 1 pound of fat, so to lose this amount, you must consume 3,500 calories fewer than you normally would[1]. Thinking in terms of losing 1pound per week, this means that if you were to eat 500 calories less per day x seven days of the week, you would have consumed 3,500 calories fewer than normal by the end of the week, which would equate to 1 pound of weight loss.

Weight Loss Math

-500 calories X 7 days = -3,500 calories = -1 pound of fat lost

As I alluded to earlier, this weight-loss process works by your body recognizing that there is a caloric shortfall, and in response, it breaks down stored fat cells in order to meet its own energy demands. If you are able to create a substantial caloric deficit day after day and week after week, it will lead to a decrease in your body's stored fat cells, which results in weight loss. Is this making sense so far? Okay, good, now we are going to add in a wrinkle to the equation: burning additional calories through exercise.

For simplicity's sake, let's continue to use the example of losing 1 pound per week by creating a caloric deficit of 500 calories per day. As we just mentioned, you can achieve this deficit by eating 500 fewer calories each day than you normally would, or you can use exercise to aid in the achievement of this deficit. For example, you could eat 250 calories less per day *and* go for a thirty-minute jog each day, during which you burn 250 calories. In this scenario, you would achieve a negative caloric balance of 500 calories per day through the combination of eating less and exercising more.

At this point, you may be thinking to yourself, instead of consuming 500 calories less per day, I'll just eat 1,000 calories less each day so that I can lose 2 pounds a week. Genius! Well, not so fast. While, in mathematical terms, this way of thinking does make sense, in fact, once you start to consider other factors such as metabolic rate and muscle loss, things become a little more complicated.

When Creating a Caloric Deficit Backfires

You may know that there are ways (which we'll discuss in more detail later on in the book) to increase your metabolism, such as through exercise and by drinking water. But you might not be aware that creating too great of a caloric deficit can slow your metabolism, thus, hindering your efforts to lose weight.

Yes, it's true that you must create a caloric deficit to lose weight; however, if that caloric deficit becomes too great, and you begin to eat less than 1,000 calories per day, it will lead to a decrease in your metabolism, which will halt weight loss and may even result in weight gain. This slow down in metabolism is caused by your body, sensing that it no longer has access to enough food to fuel its basic needs. In reaction, your body will slow your metabolism in order to conserve energy.

If, in your attempt to accelerate weight loss, you begin to eat less than 1,000 calories per day, your body will adapt, dialing back the speed of your metabolism to ensure that it has enough calories to drive basic bodily functions. When your body senses you're taking in fewer than 1,000 calories per day, it expends less energy than usual for fear that food is in scarce supply. In fact, research published in a 2016 issue of *Obesity*, which was conducted on former contestants from the television show, *The Biggest Loser*, confirmed that the body makes metabolic adjustments when you attempt to lose weight by taking extreme measures to lower your caloric intake[2]. This metabolic response actually makes a lot of sense when you put it into the context of most of human history.

Our hunter-gatherer ancestors were forced to go for long periods of time, eating fewer than 1,000 calories per day due to food insecurity. Therefore, our body's ability to slow its own metabolism in order to conserve energy probably allowed countless humans to stay alive during times of food scarcity. However, for most humans living in food-secure nations, this inherited function can lead to frustration if you are trying to lose weight by cutting your caloric intake to fewer than 1,000 calories per day, which is leading you to maintain or gain weight. In addition, eating fewer than 1,000 calories per day can also lead to a loss of muscle mass, which has been shown to slow metabolism.

When most of us think about weight loss, we are *really* thinking about fat loss. However, studies show that very-low-calorie diets, less than 1,000 calories per day, can lead to muscle loss, which can significantly slow down your metabolism[3]. Limiting yourself to 1,000 calories per day means that you'll inevitably deny yourself of important nutrients, particularly protein. When you don't eat enough protein, your body isn't supplied with the amino acids necessary to support muscle retention and growth. Even if you're exercising, your body's muscles can't be sustained or grown if they don't have the necessary protein to repair themselves. In this scenario, your body will hold onto fat, rather than muscle, because it feels as if it's starving and that it needs to keep its fat cells in reserve as an emergency energy source.

If your body is breaking down muscle cells rather than fat cells to meet its energy needs, your metabolic rate will slow. We know this to be true because it has been shown that when you are at rest, at the cellular level, one pound of fat burns only two to three calories per day, while one pound of muscle burns seven to ten calories per day. Therefore, if you took two people of the same age, gender, weight, and age, but with different amounts of muscle mass, the one with more muscle would have a faster metabolism. This is why it is important to continue to eat at least more than 1,000 calories per day so that you preserve your muscle mass and, as a result, maintain your metabolic rate.

Finding Your Sweet Spot

So far, we know that in order to lose weight, you need to create a caloric deficit significant enough for your body to use fat stores as energy. We also know that you never want to eat less than 1,000 calories per day, as this will slow your metabolism and stifle fat loss. These facts might leave you wondering, how many calories should I be eating each day in order to lose weight in a sustainable way? Well, the answer to this question will be different for everyone.

Although each individual's caloric budget is different determining the number of calories you should be eating each day to lose weight is pretty easy, due to technology. These days there are dozens of apps that will calculate your caloric budget for you, and that will allow you to easily track your caloric intake/output. Many of my patients have used *LoseIt* or *MyFitnessPal* with great success, but if you decide to track your calories, I'd recommend downloading several apps to see which is the best fit for you or reading my review on calorie-tracking apps at www.weightlostacademy.com/blog/. With that said, your plan doesn't have to include calorie tracking if you don't want it to. Remember, you are designing your own weight-loss plan, and it should only include behavioral goals that you believe in and that fit into your lifestyle

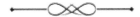

Katy: Tracking my food in a digital app on my phone turned out to be a game-changer and really taught me how to create a caloric deficit in my eating habits. I am a scientist by training, and because a digital app is essentially a data tracker, my data-loving heart took to it like a fish to water. Why do I love data? Because data doesn't lie! Data allowed me to identify trends (were there specific days/times that I was eating more or less?), correlations between behaviors (on days I had more veggies at lunch, I was much more likely to eat more veggies later in the day), and to learn exactly how to create a caloric deficit in my eating behaviors. As I've spent the past few years tracking my food (then getting out of the habit, and then restarting the habit, etc.), I have a few insights as to why logging what I'm eating to ensure a caloric deficit is so effective for my weight loss vision and goals.

First, logging my food intake gives me a <u>concrete</u> record of my food habits. Without logging my food, I have a vague idea about what I am or am not eating, but it turns out a digital record is much more reliable than my undocumented memory. It's kind of akin to having a vague idea of how much money is in my bank account versus carefully tracking my spending and/or regularly checking my account balance. The former was how I handled finances when I first struck out on my own. I had a general idea of what my paychecks were, and I had a general idea of how much money was going to rent, groceries, etc. This level of financial awareness worked okay until the day I unwittingly overdrew on my account (and by only a few dollars!). The consequence of overdrawing as a result of my "general idea" of how much money I had – a hefty bank fee – was so punishing for me that I never let it happen again. I learned to regularly track my spending and regularly check my account balance. Tracking my food allows me to similarly have an exact understanding of where I am in trying to achieve a caloric deficit instead of a "general idea" of how I'm doing calorie-wise. Prior to tracking my food regularly, I felt like I was doing pretty well eating-wise. I tried to eat healthy foods more than unhealthy foods, and that seemed okay to me. Unfortunately, the consequence of "overdrawing on my calorie budget" is not so immediately punishing as overdrawing on my bank account. It's not until I have overdrawn several days/weeks in a row that I start to realize the effects on my weight, physical functioning, and/or how my clothes are fitting. Thus, tracking my food daily provides immediate recognition when I go over my calorie budget.

The smartphone application I use for logging the food I'm eating is LoseIt, but there are a number of other options out there that do essentially the same thing. There is a huge database of foods included in the app that allows me to easily input what I am eating. I especially like the feature that allows me to use my phone to scan the barcode of an item to automatically add that item to the database for ease of entry into my food log. At the end of each day, I'm able to go back and review the foods I've eaten and analyze how that affects my calorie intake. This helps to provide the right level of awareness for me to connect what I'm eating with how many calories I'm consuming. For me, a digital platform that only requires me to type/click to input food into the log/diary is much more sustainable than keeping a pencil/paper food diary. You may decide that keeping a written food journal is more useful for you. Finding a system that works for you will be key.

So, how did I know how many calories I should be aiming for? In the app, I put in my current weight and height and then my goal weight. The app then automatically calculated the number of calories I would need to consume to lose an average of one to two pounds per week. Now, I don't live, breathe, and die by that target number, but it does give me a general idea of what I should be aiming for. I know that if I can come in just under or at that target consistently, I can achieve the one to two pound per week weight loss I'm aiming for. And that has proven to be the case for me. Knowing that a slow and steady weight loss was better for long-term health, this calculation was very helpful to me. At the beginning of every day, the app would remind me how many calories I should aim for to meet my goals. As I entered items throughout the day, the app provided a visual bar indicator showing me how much was left in my "calorie budget." Conceptually, this made a lot of sense to me, and I found it very motivating to see how many days I could meet my budget allocation without going over.

By watching the calories-consumed indicator, I became much more aware of which foods I was eating that used up a lot of my budget versus those that used fewer calories. Unsurprisingly, foods that are less nutritious eat up (pun intended) a lot more calories than more nutritious foods. I distinctly remember one day at work when a coworker announced that she had brought some birthday doughnuts to share with the office and asked if I wanted one. Instantly, I realized how much my calorie budget would be consumed if I ate one of those doughnuts. It made it much easier to turn the doughnut down so that I could "spend" those calories in other ways that day. When I wanted something sweet after dinner (a habit I developed in my early adulthood), I learned to choose a piece of fruit over a brownie because it used up so many fewer of my allotted calories. This is not to say that I never eat traditional desserts. If I know I want to eat a slice of birthday cake at a party and/or have ice-cream on a hot summer day, I simply adjust my eating elsewhere in the day, so I can accommodate my choice calorically.

Logging my food makes me accountable for my food choices **on a daily basis**. In my efforts to transform my eating habits, it has been important for me to have a daily reckoning with myself regarding the foods I decide to eat. I have a sweet tooth and, particularly when I am stressed or overwhelmed, it can be easy for me to consume foods willy-nilly with little thought for how they are impacting my body. By tracking the food I eat, I have become much more aware of how those willy-nilly eating habits have impacted the number of calories I'm consuming. When I first started logging my food, I found that I was excited about logging my food only when I knew I was going to stay within my calorie budget and/or I was meeting my wellness goals. On days when I knew I was going to go over my calorie limit, I tended to stop entering my food intake into the app, which usually only made the problem worse as I'd consume far more calories than I really wanted to. This kind of thinking is not much different from a toddler who covers his eyes and is convinced that because he can't see you, you can't see him. If I just didn't track my food, then it meant I wasn't consuming more than I should! Yeah, right.

Over time, and after many heart-to-heart moments with myself, I learned that tracking my food intake was only useful so long as I was honest with the app and, more importantly, honest with myself. I have learned that when I am going over my calorie budget, it's time to evaluate **why** I'm going over my calorie budget, and the <u>best</u> thing I can do is to <u>keep tracking</u>. By doing this, I've learned a lot about myself and my eating habits. Sometimes I ended up going over my calorie budget because I had a special event I was attending, like a birthday party or a social gathering where I ate food outside of my normal routine. Sometimes it's because I had an unexpected meal out at a restaurant (which tends to eat up calories really quickly!). But, I've learned other enlightening things about myself too. For example, I learned that when I stay up late, I tend to go over my calorie budget. When I am very stressed about a work situation, I have a tendency to consume more food. In both cases, tracking my food has allowed me to confront those behaviors and find healthier strategies to manage late nights and/or work-related stress. In this way, tracking my food intake has had direct benefits to my mental and emotional health. It's about so much more than just weight loss.

What's Next?

Creating a caloric deficit is a requirement for weight loss, although tracking your calories in order to create this deficit is not. In fact, many of my patients achieved their weight-loss goal without ever tracking their food consumption. However, all of my patients who successfully reached and sustained their weight-loss goals figured out how to create a caloric deficit while still feeling satisfied after eating. The next chapter will outline strategies on how to accomplish this.

Chapter Four Key Takeaways:

- Creating a caloric deficit is necessary for weight loss.

- You must create a caloric deficit of 3,5000 calories in order to lose one pound of fat.

- Eating fewer than 1,000 calories per day will slow your metabolism and hinder weight loss.

- Tracking your food intake and energy expenditure can help you create a caloric deficit.

Chapter 5

Achieving Satiety Through Diet

If I were asked to boil successful long-term weight loss down to one key factor, I would say that it hinges on being able to achieve satiety while eating fewer calories than normal. The eating fewer calories than normal part of this statement should already hit home with you since the previous chapter outlined why it is impossible to lose weight without creating a caloric deficit, which causes your body to use fat stores as energy. In this chapter, you'll learn how to achieve this caloric deficit without having to spend the better part of your day listening to your stomach, calling out to you for food.

Nothing can kill a weight loss plan faster than the feeling of relentless hunger. For this reason, achieving a caloric deficit, day after day for months at a time, can be challenging unless you are able to achieve satiety while eating fewer calories. There is no question that your body does not like to feel hungry, and when it does, it will send powerful messages to your brain, reminding it that you need to eat. Usually, this message comes across as something like: "STOP EVERYTHING YOU ARE DOING AND EAT! IF SOMETHING TO EAT DOESN'T COME MY WAY ANY MINUTE, I MAY NOT BE ABLE TO GO ON LIVING!! Has a message like this ever been sent from your stomach to your brain? I know that I have experienced this message being sent and that when my body is hungry enough to send this message, I've felt what seems like a primal urge to eat anything in sight as fast as I can.

You can certainly go with the option of using willpower to fight off these messages, but I wouldn't recommend this as a long-term strategy. If you are a strong-willed person, this strategy may work for a day or maybe even a week, but to employ willpower to fight off these messages over a long period of time is asking a lot of yourself. Actually, way too much, in my opinion. Therefore, in order to avoid setting yourself up to succumb to these hardcore messages and, as a result, folding on your weight-loss plan faster than the arms of a disappointed parent, it is crucial that you figure out how to achieve a caloric deficit, while at the same time achieving satiety.

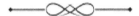

Katy: I would certainly echo the sentiment that using willpower to combat hunger is a non-sustainable long-term plan. The fact is, I just don't handle life well when I'm super hungry. Perhaps you can relate. At first, when I have them, the hunger pangs make me feel like I'm doing something "right." There is some sort of masochistic satisfaction, and my brain says, "See, look at that. I'm hungry. Go, me! There's been enough time since the last time I ate for me to feel hungry!" That feeling of self-satisfaction is generally short-lived, and I quickly morph into a different feeling that voices, "Good golly, I want to eat all the things, anything, right now because I'm SO hungry." This isn't a problem if I don't have food at my disposal. Most of the time, however, when I am in this state, I am more than willing and more than very likely to eat whatever is handy: the mints in my purse, the chocolates at my coworker's desk, the chips in the vending machine, the old package of fruit snacks I foraged from the glove box of my car . . . In my experience, this is especially the case when life gets stressful or busy – if I'm endlessly hungry **on top** of stressful situations in my life, it inevitably leads to poor decisions surrounding my food options. It has taken a lot of work, and let me assure you, this is something I'm **still** working on, but, as Ryan will discuss in the pages that follow, there are ways to set your body, mind, and environment up for success that will allow you to eat well and experience satisfaction. We'll talk through some of these in the pages that follow. If you're like me, you'll find that there are some strategies you're likely already using. I would encourage you to look for new strategies that may help revolutionize how you approach fostering success on your journey.

This may seem contradictory, but there are several strategies that you can use, which will allow you to have your cake and eat it too. But don't get too excited; eating cake is not one of the strategies. Before we learn about these strategies, it is important to first understand the process in which your body signals to your brain that it is not fully nourished and needs to consume more food.

What Does It Mean to Achieve Satiety?

Let's imagine you had a really busy morning at work. So busy, in fact, that you finally take a moment to look at the clock, which reads 2:00 p.m., and you realize that you haven't had time to eat since your 6:30

a.m. breakfast. Needless to say, you are very hungry at this point and must have something to eat before heading into your next meeting, which starts in just fifteen minutes. You contemplate heating up the soup you brought from home but decide that you just don't have the time for it. Instead, you shovel half a sleeve of crackers into your mouth while checking a few emails and then scamper down the hall to your meeting.

Just thirty minutes into your two-hour meeting, your stomach starts to rumble, calling out for you to find some nourishment. You think to yourself: "I just ate approximately 300 calories worth of crackers. Why am I already hungry? I should have just heated up my soup, but that was only 250 calories, so I guess I would have been just as hungry anyway." As your name is called out by the head of your department, your mind is forced back to business, and your stomach is left feeling helpless.

In this commonplace scenario, why wasn't your body left feeling as satisfied as it would have been if you had eaten 250 calories worth of soup instead of eating 300 calories worth of crackers? To answer this question, we must examine the interactions between your stomach and your brain. Your stomach is the receptor of everything you ingest, and one of its primary responsibilities is to signal to your brain that what it has ingested has triggered satiety.

Satiety, the sensation that you've eaten enough to feel full, results when your body achieves a balance of hormonal and neurological signals reaching your brain from your stomach. As you might expect, satiety results when a certain volume of food is ingested. The feeling of satiety is transmitted from your stomach to your brain by an automatic feedback mechanism.

When your body reaches satiety, your stomach signals to your brain to stop eating. One mechanism that triggers this signal comes as a result of your stomach wall stretching to accommodate the meal you are eating. When your stomach wall expands, nerve stretch receptors send signals to the brain that the stomach is expanding and that you can begin to taper off and stop eating. At the same time this stomach stretching is taking place, a hormone called ghrelin, produced when your stomach empties to trigger a hunger message, starts to decrease. This drop in ghrelin causes the number of signals reaching your brain, which are telling it to stop eating, to outnumber the signals which are encouraging your brain to continue eating; as a result, your brain recognizes that you have reached satiety.

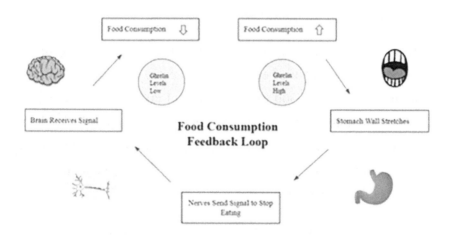

Food Consumption Feedback Loop

Now that you understand the process of achieving satiety, let's talk about the strategies you can use to reach satiety while losing weight. The two primary strategies to use in order to feel satisfied while achieving a caloric deficit center around food volume and the rate of digestion. Under these two umbrella strategies, we will go into depth about "volumetrics," water intake, and food composition. Also, within this section, we will discuss secondary yet important behavioral strategies for achieving satiety.

Strategies for Achieving Satiety

If your stomach signals your brain to stop eating when the stomach wall is stretched to a certain point, then it is logical to hypothesize that the amount of food you eat is an important part of achieving satiety. Dr. Barbara Rolls, head of Nutritional Sciences at Pennsylvania State University, spent years researching this hypothesis, which led to the development of the concept of *Volumetrics*[1].

Through her research, Dr. Rolls discovered that your body is wired to feel full based on the volume of food that you eat. In fact, she has observed that over the course of a day or two, a person will consistently eat about the same weight of the food. Therefore, Dr. Rolls was able to determine that if a person can lower the number of calories they are eating while maintaining the consumption of the same total volume of food, they will be able to lose weight without having to feel like they are starving themselves.

The key to eating the same volume of food while reducing the number of calories is to consume foods that contain high amounts of water and fiber. These types of foods include fruits, vegetables, and whole grains. As an example, let's return to our scenario of having to choose between eating 250 calories worth of soup or 300 calories worth of crackers for lunch.

In the original example, you chose to eat the crackers rather than take the time to heat up your soup, which left you feeling hungry just a short time later because crackers contain very little water and fiber and, as a result, not very filling. If you were to play this scenario out further, you would probably end up eating more crackers as soon as the meeting was over because you were still really hungry. In this case, by the time you would have consumed enough crackers to stretch your stomach and signal to your brain that you are full and that you can stop eating, you would have ended up eating 600 calories worth of crackers (300 calories before the meeting and 300 calories after the meeting).

But what if you were to rewind and decided instead to take the extra time to heat up your soup and eat it before your meeting? Well, your vegetable soup is high in fiber and water, so it would have caused your stomach wall to stretch out enough to signal to your brain that you are satisfied and can stop eating. As a result, you would end up going to your meeting feeling nice and full and probably wouldn't have felt the urge to eat again until you arrive home for dinner. Leaving you satiated and with a caloric lunch total of only 250 calories.

In both scenarios, you ended up eating the right volume of food to stretch your stomach enough to signal satiety. However, by choosing to eat the vegetable soup, which was high in fiber and water, you were able to eat a satisfying lunch that was only 250 calories vs. the 600 calories worth of crackers it took to make you feel full. This comes out to a net difference of 350 calories, which in isolation isn't that meaningful, but if you were to apply this principle of volumetrics to all of your meals, you can see how it would very rapidly help you lose weight without having to feel the pain of extreme hunger. In addition to the amount of food you consume, leading to satiety, the volume of food that you *view* prior to eating can make a difference in how full you feel after eating.

A number of studies have demonstrated that the perceived size of a food product is an important factor related to satiety[2]. The information gathered from these studies suggests that at least a portion of the information about the satiating potential of a meal is gathered by your body before you even start eating. For instance, if a person has a small cookie placed in front of them that is 150 calories and then eats it, the chances are that they won't feel very full after. However, if a large bowl of salad that is also 150 calories is placed in front of that same person, they are much more likely to feel satisfied after eating it. This is, of course, because the weight/volume of a cookie is minimal compared to the salad and because our brains visually interpret eating a large portion of food as leading to satiety, regardless of how many calories the food contains. Now that you have a handle on how your body can become satiated while consuming fewer calories than you normally do, let's learn about what types of foods you can eat that will keep you feeling satisfied for hours on end.

Strategies for Maintaining Satiety

Satiety's Big Three – Fiber, Water, and Protein

The term "the big three" refers to the most prominent entities in any given grouping or subject. Memorable big three's in recent history include World War II's big three: the United States, Great Britain, and the Soviet Union; broadcast television's big three: ABC, CBS, and NBC; the Boston Celtic's big three of the 1980s: Larry Bird, Kevin Mchale, and Robert Parish, and of course "This Is Us's" big three: Randall, Kate, and Kevin. In the world of achieving satiety while losing weight, the big three refers to fiber, water, and protein.

By eating a diet rich in fiber, water, and protein, you are able to delay gastric emptying, which is the rate at which food passes through your stomach. With this delay, you will be able to feel full longer, which will make you less likely to be looking for snacks in between meals. In contrast, if you were to eat a diet that is high in simple starches or sugars, this would result in rapid gastric emptying and subsequent routine hunger.

When you digest simple starches (white bread products, white rice, white pasta, etc.) and sugars (crackers, cookies, fruit juices, etc.), they move rapidly through your stomach and into your bloodstream. This fast-paced transmission creates a spike in your blood sugar, which causes your pancreas to secrete insulin in order to keep your blood sugar levels in a healthy range. When insulin is released into your bloodstream, it stimulates muscle, fat, and liver cells to absorb the sugar within your blood, known as glucose. The cells can use this glucose for energy, but if it is not needed for energy, the excess glucose is converted into fat cells for long-term storage. This is why a diet that is high in sugars, which are quickly digested, can lead to the creation of excess fat cells. When this cycle is repeated on a consistent basis, it can lead to significant weight gain.

The good news is that if you are able to eat a diet composed predominantly of the big three and limited simple starches, you will be able to maintain a slow rate of gastric emptying. This delayed gastric emptying will keep you feeling full longer and will help you avoid spikes in your blood sugar, which leads to the storage of excess fat cells. To better understand why the big three are so important to a successful weight loss plan, let's examine each of them individually.

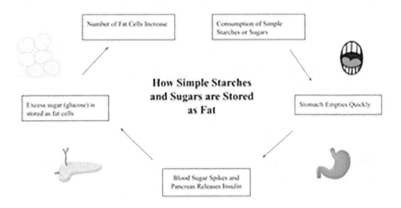

Figure: How Simple Starches and Sugars are Stored as Fat — cycle diagram with the following elements: Number of Fat Cells Increase; Consumption of Simple Starches or Sugars; Stomach Empties Quickly; Blood Sugar Spikes and Pancreas Releases Insulin; Excess sugar (glucose) is stored as fat cells.

Fiber

If I were to try to sell you something that you could eat that would make you feel full for hours but contained absolutely no calories, you'd probably think I was trying to scam you, or you'd laugh me out of the room. But this magical food component does, in fact, exist and it's called fiber.

Fiber is a common macronutrient that you eat, but that is not digestible by your body. Since fiber is not digestible, it remains in your stomach for long periods of time. While fiber is sitting in your stomach, it soaks up water and expands just like a sponge. As you now know, when your stomach expands, it pushes on nerve receptors, which signal to the brain that it is full and that you should taper eating. By helping to expand the stomach and by slowing gastric emptying, fiber helps you achieve and maintain satiety for long stretches of time. You can find large amounts of fiber in foods like whole grains, legumes, fruits, and vegetables.

Unlike simple starches, grains found in foods like whole-wheat bread products, whole-grain cereal, whole-wheat pasta, brown rice, and potatoes, when consumed with the skin, offer large amounts of fiber per serving. Similarly, legumes, a plant that produces a pod with seeds inside it, also contain high levels of fiber. Common legumes include lentils, peas, chickpeas, beans, soybeans, peas, edamame, lentils, and beans. Please see the table below for some examples of whole grains and legumes that are high in fiber.

Whole Grains	Fiber per serving (g)	Legumes	Fiber per serving (g)
All-Bran, Kelloggs	10.0	Pinto Beans	14.7
Whole Wheat Pasta	6.3	Baked Beans	14.0
Baked Potato	5.0	Lima Beans	13.2
Brown Rice	3.5	Peas	4.0
Whole Wheat Bread	2.0	Green Beans	2.0

There is a good chance that you've heard that eating five servings of fruits and vegetables a day can help to promote weight loss. Well, one of the reasons this is true is because fruits and vegetables offer large amounts of fiber and contain few calories. Nearly every type of fruit and vegetable offers some amount of fiber, so there is no wrong choice, but here are the top five fruits and vegetables in regard to the amount of fiber they contain[3]:

Fruits	Fiber per serving (g)	Vegetables	Fiber per serving (g)
Raspberries	8.4	Artichokes	6.2
Blueberries	4.0	Beets	3.8
Pears	4.0	Squash	3.0
Apples	3.7	Broccoli	2.3
Strawberries	3.4	Spinach	2.2

The daily recommended intake of fiber is 25 grams for women and 38 grams for men. If you are able to reach these daily recommendations, it will certainly help to keep you feeling satisfied throughout the day, especially when combined with adequate water intake.

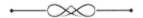

Katy: As I was learning how to adjust the foods I was eating to better support my overall health, one of the decisions I made was to try to eat fewer boxed or processed foods. I didn't specify or quantify exactly what that meant, but I simply started with trying to eat just a little less processed foods. What that unwittingly led to was a substantial increase in the amount of fiber I consumed. So, what did this look like? Prior to this decision, the following things were regular staples in my diet: boxed macaroni and cheese, ramen noodles, instant pasta kits (hamburger helper, pasta-roni), freezer meals like chicken pot pie, burritos, and pizza, crackers, chips, etc. I did not eliminate all of these things at once (heavens, I would have mutinied against myself if I'd done that!). I started small and made incremental changes over the course of several weeks, months, and years. I don't remember exactly what I decided to eliminate first, but I think it might have been the instant pasta kits. I was well aware that not only were these kits comprised of simple carbohydrates, but there were other additives I didn't necessarily want in my body either. So, if I was eliminating these simple carbohydrates and processed foods, what was I eating instead?? I started by making some homemade soups (I really got to know my crockpot well) and revisited recipes my mom had made when I was growing up. These weren't always the picture of health (I remember more than one very buttery, creamy soup in the rotation), but I started altering what I was eating. And for me, choosing homemade items (i.e., less processed) was a step toward slowly increasing things like my fiber intake. I tried things I wasn't used to eating: I made homemade beans (not a favorite) and lentils (which I loved, but my body had a hard time processing at first). I started finding substitutes for pasta like spaghetti squash, zucchini noodles, and/or cauliflower rice. I really have come to love these options because not only do they help satisfy a pasta craving, but I'm getting added fiber because of the veggies. I count that as a win-win situation.

Now, in full disclosure, it's important to note that I still eat pasta on occasion (I went to Italy a couple of summers ago and gladly partook in the absolutely delicious fresh pasta), and sometimes I still eat pizza (again, in Italy? Yes, please! But, sometimes I eat pizza when I'm **not** in Italy too.). From the beginning, it has always been important to me that I still enjoy my life, and the truth is, sometimes, that involves eating the pasta (especially when in Italy). The important principle for me to internalize; however, has been to recognize and be intentional about those food items I want to be part of my regular eating routine. If I'm regularly consuming fruits, vegetables, whole grains, and other foods with good amounts of fiber, that significantly increases the likelihood that I will consume the appropriate amount of calories my body needs to maintain a healthy weight.

Water

Like fiber, water offers a zero-calorie way to ensure that you reach satiety when eating and maintain a feeling of satisfaction throughout the day. Numerous studies have shown that drinking water may promote weight loss and weight maintenance[4]. Staying well-hydrated can enhance weight-loss results by helping your body to achieve satiety and by increasing your metabolic rate.

Believe it or not, it is very difficult for your body to make the distinction between whether or not it is hungry or thirsty. As a result, you often end up giving your body food when, in reality, it is in need of water. Therefore, staying well hydrated is an easy way to ensure that your body is getting what it is asking for while avoiding excess calorie consumption. In addition to fulfilling your primal need to stay hydrated, drinking plenty of water before meals has been shown to help people reach satiety while taking in fewer calories.

Research has shown that drinking a glass of water right before a meal helps you to feel more full and eat less. The mechanism for this is pretty straightforward. If you recall, the previous section on "volumetrics" explained that your stomach would send a signal to your brain when it is stretched to a certain point, indicating that it is full and that you should stop eating. If you drink water before or during your meal, it will take up room in your stomach, stretching it and causing it to alert your brain that it is full. This simple act of drinking water before each meal can have a significant impact on weight loss.

Studies that have looked at the effect of water consumption before meals in middle-aged and older adults have displayed a meaningful change in weight. These studies indicate that drinking water before each meal may increase weight loss by three to four pounds in over just a twelve-week period[5,6]. Specifically, one such study examined middle-aged overweight and obese individuals who drank water before each meal, compared to a group that did not drink water before meals. The study found that the group who drank water before each meal, over twelve weeks, lost 44 percent more weight compared to the group who did not[6]. Not only is drinking water a powerful way to increase satiety while avoiding an increase in caloric consumption, but it can also increase your metabolic rate.

Your metabolic rate, or the speed of your metabolism, is the rate or the speed at which your body burns calories while at rest. The consistent consumption of water has been shown to increase your metabolic rate, which can lead to weight loss[7,8]. The uptick in your metabolic rate after drinking water is caused by your body expending energy to internally heat the water. After drinking cold water, your body needs to heat it up to its own internal temperature. Just like your hot water heater needs the energy to warm up water for you to take a nice hot shower, your own body needs to expend energy in order to heat up water that you drink. The energy to warm up this water comes from your body's fat stores. Breaking down fat stores to use as energy causes an increase in your metabolic rate, and when done over and over again, this process can lead to weight loss.

The concept of harnessing water to increase your metabolic rate has been put to the test in several studies. In two notable studies, adults' resting metabolic rate was shown to increase by 24 to 30 percent within ten minutes of drinking water. These studies showed that this increase in metabolic rate lasted for at least sixty minutes after the water was consumed[7,8]. Another study of overweight women examined the effects of increasing water intake to 34 ounces or just over four cups of water per day. The researchers found that over a twelve-month period, this increase in water consumption resulted in an extra 4.4 pounds of weight loss[9]. In my opinion, since the women who took part in this study didn't make any lifestyle changes except to drink more water, these results are significant. As you can see, increasing your water consumption and drinking water prior to meals can serve as a catalyst for satiety, an increase in your metabolic rate, and subsequent weight loss. The same is true for the third member of our big three, protein.

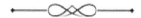

Katy: I have always been a water, milk, and sometimes juice kind of person. I have never particularly enjoyed soda (primarily because of the carbonation, I think), and I don't drink alcohol or coffee, so water is often what I choose anyway, simply because I prefer it. I know that is not the case for everyone. I have very dear family members that <u>much</u> prefer soda to other beverages and/or can only stomach water when it is enhanced with flavors and/or infused with lemons, limes, or cucumbers. I can appreciate the challenge it would be to get enough water if your mouth, brain, and body are crying out for a flavor of some kind. In that case, I think choosing flavor enhancers such as lemons and limes are a great option.

This is not to say that getting enough water has always been a picnic for me. My issue with getting enough water? I find it irritating how much it interrupts my daily schedule to constantly be running to the bathroom! Not only is it a hassle, but sometimes it is just not feasible. I am a college professor, and it is impractical to have to leave in the middle of teaching a class just to use the bathroom. That said, I have learned that my bladder urges do eventually level off and get used to increased water intake. Perhaps yours will too? And, besides, flushing my kidneys regularly is an added health benefit, too, right? Although drinking enough water is something that I have definitely gotten better at, I still struggle some days to get in an adequate amount of water to help contribute to feelings of satiety. Keeping refillable water bottles handy (in my car, at my desk, on my kitchen counter) has helped immensely. I know that to drink the amount of water I'm aiming for, I need to drink the equivalent of filling my favorite water bottle four times over.

Protein

If the Big Three were to have a team captain, it would surely be protein. Protein would undoubtedly be the captain of "team satiety" because of the considerable experimental and real-world research, which shows that increasing the amount of protein in your diet without changing the number of calories you consume can lead to enhanced feelings of satiety[2]. Protein is so effective at helping you achieve satiety because it reduces your hunger hormones and increases the levels of the hormones that make you feel full.

As you may recall, ghrelin is a hormone that travels from your digestive system through your bloodstream and, eventually, your brain, alerting it that you are hungry and that you better start searching for food. As a result, as the levels of ghrelin in your bloodstream rise, so does your appetite. This increase in appetite causes you to eat more food, take in more calories, and store more fat. The good news is that eating protein can result in a reduction in ghrelin levels, which can lead to a reduction in caloric consumption and subsequent weight loss.

In a study that examined healthy adults, half of the participants were fed a breakfast high in protein, while the other half were fed a breakfast high in carbohydrates. When the researchers measured ghrelin levels through a blood test, after participants finished eating, they found that the group that ate the high protein breakfast had much lower levels of ghrelin when compared to the group that ate the high carbohydrate breakfast[10]. In addition to lowering levels of ghrelin, eating protein can also increase levels of peptide YY, a hormone that makes you feel full.

Peptide YY is a hormone that is released from your digestive system in response to eating and alerts your brain that you are satiated and should stop eating. Research has shown that high-protein intake induces the greatest release of peptide YY and the most pronounced feelings of satiety when compared to eating carbohydrates or fats[11]. As you can imagine, this effect of increasing the amount of the hormone that alerts your brain that you are full (peptide YY) while at the same time reducing the amount of hormone that tells your brain that it is hungry (ghrelin) is a wonderful recipe for reaching satiety. Furthermore, this feeling of satiety from eating protein lasts for long periods of time due to slow rates of gastric emptying.

I can remember as a child not enjoying eating large portions of meat because it took so much energy to chew the meat to the point of making it ready to be swallowed. It was especially compared to how easy it was to chew through a piece of pasta. I bet our stomach feels the same way when it comes to digesting protein. Breaking down protein so it can be absorbed into the bloodstream is a complex process, a process that is much lengthier than the digestion of carbohydrates. As a result, protein remains in your stomach, just like it remained in my mouth as a child, for much longer periods of time when compared to other macronutrients.

This extended digestive period associated with protein, along with the reduction in ghrelin and increase in peptide YY, is why protein is able to keep you feeling satisfied for much longer. When protein finally fully breaks down, it is absorbed into your bloodstream without triggering an insulin response. As you may recall, when you absorb foods that are high in sugar (glucose) like simple starches, your blood glucose levels spike, causing your pancreas to release insulin, which causes glucose to be transported to your cells in order to be stored as fat. Due to protein's positive effect on hunger hormones, its slow digestion rate, and its inability to cause an insulin response, eating a diet rich in protein has been linked to weight loss and healthy weight maintenance. In order to maximize the benefit of a protein-rich diet, it is best to stick to lean protein sources and avoid protein sources that are high in saturated fats. Here are some lean protein sources that you might like to consider incorporating into your diet:

Lean Protein	Protein per serving (g)	Saturated fat per serving (g)
Turkey Breast	24	2
Solid White Tuna	20	.5
Chicken Breast	19	.9
Salmon	17	2.6
Greek Yogurt (non-fat)	17	0

Cottage Cheese (non-fat)	14	0
Egg	6	1.6

*a serving of meat is 3 ounces

*a serving of Greek yogurt is 6 ounces

*a serving of cottage cheese is 4 ounces

Katy: Getting enough protein is, for me, an ongoing challenge. Most of this has to do with the planning it requires to make sure I have good options. Some of my most reliable go-to protein sources have been hard-boiled eggs, jerky (but I try to watch how much sugar they add to it!), cottage cheese, and tuna packets.

Although not part of the Big Three, if we were to add an honorable mention to the group, it would have to be "good" fats.

For a Weight Lost tip sheet that details the "3 Steps to Creating Satiating Meals" that incorporate the Big Three, please visit https://weightlostacademy.com/home-2/resources/

Eating Fat to Lose Fat

If the macronutrient fat was to disclose its relationship status on social media, it would read, "it's complicated." Fat is a complex nutrient because, on the one hand, there are certain fats, namely unsaturated and trans fats, that are just not good for you. Consumption of these types of fats over time can lead to weight gain and heart disease. However, on the other hand, there are other types of fats, polyunsaturated and monounsaturated, or "good fats," that can help to lower your risk for heart disease and can, in fact, help you lose weight by increasing feelings of satiety.

Over the years, dietary fat has developed a reputation as the enemy to weight loss. This reputation is well deserved for saturated and trans fats, which have been linked to obesity, high cholesterol, and heart disease. However, polyunsaturated and monounsaturated fats, otherwise known as "good fats," have been shown to lower bad cholesterol, increase good cholesterol, and reduce your risk for developing heart disease. Additionally, these fats have been shown to inhibit the emptying of food from the stomach, keeping you feeling full for longer periods of time[12].

Like protein, fats digest more slowly than carbohydrates. This slow digestion rate increases gastric emptying time, which in turn prolongs the length of time that you feel satisfied after eating. Although fats carry more than double the calories of protein, nine calories per one gram, as compared to four calories per one gram of protein, choosing to selectively eat "good fats" can help to promote weight loss by increasing satiety. Ideally, it is best to select foods that are high in "good fats" and low in saturated fats. Here are some examples of foods that you may consider incorporating into your diet that offers high amounts of good fats:

Sources of 'good fats"	"Good Fats" per serving (g)	Saturated fat per serving (g)
Avocados	23.7	4.3

Olive Oil	11.4	1.9
Salmon	6.7	2.6
Flaxseed	3.8	.4

*a serving of olive oil and flaxseed is 1 tablespoon

*a serving of salmon is 3 ounces

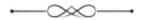

Katy: I am so glad for the shift in popular thinking when it comes to healthy fats. I try to always have some on hand in my pantry and refrigerator because they are so satiating. Some of my go-to healthy fats: green olives, avocados, and nuts.

By this point, we've discussed fiber, protein, and good fats, which may leave you wondering why I haven't mentioned nuts or nut butter. Well, because nuts are a good source of fiber, protein, and good fats, I thought they deserved their very own section.

Nuts: Weight Loss Superfood

At first glance, nuts may look like a weight-loss goal killer as they contain a ton of calories in a relatively small serving size. However, if you dig deeper, you'll find that nuts are chalked full of fiber, protein, and healthy fats, which, as you know, are the key nutrients that keep us feeling full and, as a result, promote weight loss. In fact, the research shows that nuts may be one of if not the best type of food you can eat to promote weight loss.

There are many research studies that suggest that consuming nuts on a regular basis can help you lose weight [13, 14, 15, 16, 17]. In one such study, researchers took sixty-five overweight or obese individuals and split them into two groups. The first group ate a low-calorie diet supplemented with almonds and the second group ate a low-calorie diet supplemented with complex carbohydrates. Both groups consumed equal amounts of calories, protein, cholesterol, and saturated fat. At the end of a twenty-four-week period, the group who supplemented their diet with almonds had a 62 percent greater reduction in weight and body mass index (BMI), a 50 percent greater reduction in waist circumference, and a 56 percent greater reduction in fat mass[18]. A leading theory behind why nuts help to promote weight loss is that they increase feelings of satiety.

Research studies have shown that adding nuts to your diet has been linked to feelings of reduced hunger and feeling full for longer periods of time[19,20]. In fact, research suggests that around fifty to 100 percent of the extra calories that come from introducing nuts into your diet are canceled out by a natural reduction in the intake of other foods[21,22]. In other words, snacking on nuts increases feelings of satiety, which results in eating less of other types of foods, which can lead to the achievement of a caloric deficit and future weight loss[23].

Okay, you got it, right? Nuts are a little powerhouse of food that can help you feel full for long periods of time and, as a result, have been shown to lead to weight loss. So, what type of nuts should you eat in order to lose weight? The simple answer is all of them.

Almost all nuts have high amounts of fiber, protein, and good fats, so it is hard to go wrong choosing which types of nuts to consume. Ideally, it is best to eat a variety of nuts; however, I'd recommend that you use your discretion to decide which nuts to consume based on your pallet and budget. Here are the nutrition facts on the most commonly consumed nuts:

Nut	Protein per serving (g)	Fiber per serving (g)	"Good fats" per serving (g)
Peanuts	7	2.4	11.4
Almonds	6	4	12.5
Cashews	5	.9	9.2
Walnuts	4.3	1.9	15.5
Pecans	2.6	2.7	18
*all one-ounce servings			

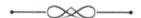

Katy: Nuts have been a really helpful part of my eating plan. First off, as Ryan points out, they are a solid, healthy fat that can really contribute to a feeling of satiety. From a practical standpoint, one of the reasons I love nuts is because they are portable, and they satisfy the snacking urge for me. It sounds so silly, but the truth is, I have grown accustomed to eating pieces of things in stages – like chips, M&Ms, popcorn, etc. Eating nuts has been a really helpful alternative to help satisfy that piecemeal snack craving. My one caution: some nuts come salted, seasoned, and/or coated in chocolate. Make sure you're not negating the benefits of the nuts themselves as a result of what they're covered in.

As you can see, the type of foods that you eat and, in turn, the underlying macronutrients you consume are major factors when it comes to achieving satiety. By choosing foods that are rich in water, fiber, protein, and good fats, you will be able to achieve satiety while reducing the total calories you consume. This way of eating can lead to sustainable weight-loss results because it allows you to consistently create a caloric deficit without feeling like you are starving yourself.

What's Next?

Although eating the right types of foods is a critically important piece of achieving satiety while consuming fewer calories, there are other behavioral factors that are major players in the achievement of satiety. These behaviors include how often you are eating, how much you are sleeping, and how you are approaching breakfast. These behaviors will be the focus of the next chapter.

Chapter Five Key Takeaways:

- Achieving satiety when eating is crucial to achieving sustainable weight loss.

- Fiber contains no calories but makes you feel full – females are recommended to eat at least twenty-five grams per day and males thirty-eight grams per day.

- Staying hydrated increases feelings of satiety – drinking a glass of water before and/or during a meal has been shown to promote weight loss.

- Consuming lean protein and good fats have been shown to increase satiety and promote weight loss.

- Nuts are a good source of fiber, protein, and good fat and have been shown to promote weight loss.

Chapter 6

Achieving Satiety Through Daily Habits

It doesn't take Sherlock Holmes to be able to see that there is a connection between the amount and types of foods you eat and satiety. However, there are less obvious behavioral choices you make every day that affect your body's feelings of hunger and satisfaction. Three of the behavioral habits that have been closely linked to achieving satiety are: how often you eat (meal frequency), how much and how well you sleep, and what you are choosing to eat for breakfast.

These behaviors will contribute to how hungry you feel throughout the day, how often you are looking for something to eat, and how satisfied you feel after eating. In order to help you determine if changing your approach(es) to meal frequency, sleep, and breakfast is something you'd like to make a part of your weight-loss plan, we will look at each one of these behaviors and their relationship to satiety, in depth. Let's start by examining meal frequency.

Meal Frequency: Harnessing Your Ancient DNA

If there is one thing our bodies are trained to do well, it is to eat when we feel hungry. This should come as no surprise if you consider human evolution. Our genes have been evolving for hundreds of millions of years, and for 99.9 percent of our evolution, these genes have been developing in an environment of food insecurity. As a result, our brains have evolved to interpret feelings of hunger as a precursor to death, and the feeling of satiety as something that leads to the continuation of life.

Although our ability to mass-produce and store food has greatly changed over the last several hundred years, our genetics have not. Our bodies still have several mechanisms in place to ensure that we remember to eat. For the vast majority of our existence, these mechanisms helped humans live through long periods of time when food was unavailable.

For example, let's imagine that one of your ancient ancestors was fortunate enough to have killed a wildebeest during a hunt. This ancestor's brain instructed him to continue to eat the meat as long as it was available to him, as, without modern refrigeration, it was sure to spoil in short order. This instruction from his brain allowed your ancestor to eat many, many more calories of the wildebeest meat than he needed for energy at that time, which resulted in his body storing these extra calories as fat cells. This message sent from your ancestor's brain that encouraged him to overeat in order to store excess calories as fat cells literally was a lifesaver: It would have been quite common for this same ancestor to endure long periods of time when there wasn't enough food to eat. During these periods, your ancestor's body would break down his stored fat cells to use as energy in order to keep his vital organs running and quite literally keep him alive and breathing.

Bringing us back to the modern-day, the mechanism that tells you to over-consume food if you are hungry has not changed and is, therefore, still part of your genetic makeup. However, as we know, in developed countries there is more than enough food available for people to eat all of the time. As a consequence of humans' recent ability to mass-produce and store food, this genetic mechanism that triggers people to overeat when they are hungry has been rendered obsolete. Unfortunately, rather than this mechanism keeping you alive as it did for your ancestors, it is promoting the storage of excess fat cells, which results in weight gain.

In order for you to avoid calling upon this ancient mechanism that makes you over-consume food and stores excess fat cells, it is best for you to avoid becoming overly hungry. We've all been at the point where we feel like we are "starving" and can feel this mechanism being triggered within us. What takes place after this mechanism is set off isn't very pretty. Typically, what happens next is a melee to eat anything and everything you can find, no matter the nutritional content, until your body tells you that it has consumed enough food to feel satiated. Once this primal need has been met, you often don't feel great about what types of foods you ate and how much you consumed. But this type of reaction to feeling overly hungry can be avoided by keeping yourself feeling satisfied but not overly full.

A typical American eating routine often consists of a small or nonexistent breakfast, lunch, dinner, and some post-dinner snacking. For some people, this type of eating schedule works just fine. However, the majority of Americans are overweight or obese, which can lead to the assumption that this type of eating routine doesn't promote the maintenance of a healthy weight, let alone weight loss[1]. One reason this might be true is that going for long periods of time within the day without eating can trigger your body's mechanism to overeat.

One way to try to avoid triggering our ancient mechanism to overconsume is to eat small meals or snacks every three to four hours. If these meals and snacks are appropriately portioned, this frequency of eating will allow your body to feel satiated throughout the day, which will help you avoid feelings of excess hunger that signal your body to eat more food than it needs. This simple approach of deliberately eating every few hours will allow you to make rational food choices based on your values, goals, and the nutritional content of the food.

Of course, it is essential to create an eating schedule that works best for you when considering your other obligations throughout the day and what types of food and/or food storage options you have available to you. However, to get you thinking about what type of plan might work best for you, here is a sample eating routine that incorporates frequent meals and snacks:

Type of Food	Time
Breakfast	7:00 a.m.
Morning snack	10:00 a.m.
Lunch	1:00 p.m.
Afternoon snack	4:00 p.m.
Dinner	6:30 p.m.

This sample-eating schedule gives you an idea of how often you might want to consider eating in order to avoid feelings of extreme hunger throughout the day. As you probably noticed, eating breakfast is included in this sample plan. Next, we'll examine breakfast and how the type of foods you eat in the morning can affect your ability to feel satiated and lose weight.

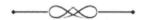

Katy: Making sure I plan my day so that I don't get too hungry has been an essential part of my eating plan. I grew up in a home that had set meal times, but as I got older, I had free access to the kitchen at any time of the day, evening, or night. This meant that not only was I eating at mealtimes, but I was also eating in between, effectively grazing for most of the day. When I moved out on my own, my eating became more erratic and unpredictable. I would either graze throughout the day or because of school and work commitments, I would go several hours without eating anything at all, only to eat large amounts of food when I finally had time. Either option was not working for my health or my weight. As my life and work schedule has become more predictable, it has allowed me to have a more predictable and plan-able eating schedule. I believe that it's important to recognize that your eating plan might look slightly different than someone else's, but by implementing the general principles that do your body good, you can find something that works for you. For me, it changes depending on what my schedule is. Here's what I have found to work for me:

On days when I teach an early class:

- ✓ Breakfast at 7:00 a.m.
- ✓ Snack around 10:30 a.m.
- ✓ Lunch around 1:00 p.m.
- ✓ Snack around 4:00 p.m.
- ✓ Dinner around 6:00 or 6:30 p.m.
- ✓ The kitchen is closed after 8:00 p.m.

On days when I don't have to be to work until about 9:00 a.m., my eating schedule looks slightly different:

- ✓ Breakfast around 8:30 a.m.
- ✓ Lunch around 12:30 p.m.
- ✓ Snack around 3:30 p.m.
- ✓ Dinner around 6:30 or 7:00 p.m.
- ✓ The kitchen is closed after 8:00 p.m.

On weekends, my eating schedule looks different in other ways!

- ✓ Snack before I head out hiking/biking/some other form of exercise around 7 :00 or 8 :00 a.m.
- ✓ Brunch around 10:00 a.m.
- ✓ Lunch around 2:00 p.m.
- ✓ Dinner around 6:30 or 7:00 p.m.
- ✓ The kitchen is closed after 8:00 p.m.

These are not set in stone but are general rules of thumb that I follow for my eating plans. Importantly, I have made a guideline for myself that the kitchen is closed after 8 :00 p.m. What does this mean? It means no eating/snacking/grazing after 8:00 p.m. This has turned out to be a rather pivotal decision in my overall health. Before I made this decision, I found that I was a habitual late-night snacker. While I was watching TV or a movie, reading a book, or chatting on the phone, I was just simply in the habit of snacking after dinner. Once I cut out late-night snacking, I started consuming far fewer calories. And, let's be honest, it's not like I was giving up healthy snacks like carrot sticks and hummus by stopping eating by 8 p.m. My nighttime snacks were almost exclusively foods that were definitely not contributing to healthy eating habits.

Breakfast: Still the Most Important Meal of the Day . . . with a Catch

We've all heard the old cliché "breakfast is the most important meal of the day." Throughout your lifetime, I bet you've heard this phrase directed your way with the implication that it is a nutritional fact from various people like: a parent, doctor, teacher, and maybe even your spouse. What you might not know is this phrase was born during a 1944 marketing campaign by General Foods, then the makers of Grape Nuts, in order to sell more cereal. While this slogan may have helped promote cereal, it left a misconception about breakfast in its wake, especially when it comes to weight loss.

Research has shown that eating breakfast does not alone help people lose weight. In fact, studies show that eating just any type of breakfast can add extra calories to your diet, which may result in weight gain[2]. However, studies also show that eating a breakfast that is high in protein can have the opposite effect.

Assuming you read the previous section on protein consumption and weight loss, this concept should not come as much of a surprise. Adding more protein to your diet is a proven way to achieve weight loss as it can increase your feelings of satiety, which helps to curb your appetite and keeps you from overeating. In fact, studies have shown that eating a high-protein breakfast has been shown to reduce hunger and help people eat up to 135 fewer calories throughout the day[3,4,5]. Research suggests that this reduction in hunger and caloric intake from eating a protein-rich breakfast may be linked to changes in brain signaling and hormone levels.

Circling back to our previous learning, we know that consuming protein helps you curb your appetite by reducing the production of ghrelin, the hormone that increases appetite and increases your production of peptide YY, the hormone that increases satiety. Studies have found that starting your day with a breakfast rich in protein can affect these hormones throughout the day, which can lead to increases in satiety and a reduction in overall caloric intake[6,7,8]. Increasing your feelings of satiety by eating a protein-based breakfast instead of a grain-based breakfast has been shown to lead to weight loss when this habit is measured over time.

A study of obese Chinese teens showed that replacing a grain-based breakfast with an egg-based meal led to significantly more weight loss over three months. The higher-protein breakfast group lost 3.9 percent of their body weight or 5.3 pounds, while the lower-protein group lost only 0.2 percent or 0.2 pounds[9]. In a similar study, people on a weight loss program received either an egg breakfast or a bagel breakfast with the same amount of calories. After eight weeks, those eating the egg breakfast had a 61 percent higher reduction in BMI, 65 percent more weight loss, and a 34 percent greater reduction in waist measurements, as compared to the group who ate the bagel breakfast[10].

This body of research indicates that eating a protein-rich breakfast has the ability to help promote weight loss when instituted as a sustainable behavior change. With this knowledge under your belt, I'd like you to consider adopting a new slogan when it comes to breakfast: "a *high-protein* breakfast is the most important meal of the day." Although the amount of protein consumed for breakfast was variable across these research studies, if you decide to incorporate a protein-rich breakfast into your lifestyle, I would recommend aiming for at least 15 grams of protein each morning. Here are some examples of what types of foods you may incorporate to reach this goal:

Breakfast 1: *A cup of oatmeal made with skim milk and almonds= 20 grams of protein*

Breakfast 2: *Two eggs on a whole-wheat English muffin= 17 grams of protein*

Breakfast 3: *Non-fat Greek yogurt with your favorite fruit mixed in=* *17 grams of protein*

> To download the *Weight Lost: High Protein and Fiber Breakfast Recipe Guide* for free, please visit
> https://weightlostacademy.com/home-2/resources/

Of course, I would recommend adding fruits and vegetables to all of these meal options in order to create a meal that is high in protein but also incorporates good fats and fiber. Now that we have a good handle on how to incorporate protein into your morning routine let's turn our attention to the very important behavior that has a meaningful impact on satiety and takes place just before you consume breakfast. Yes, you guessed it, this habit is sleep.

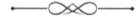

Katy: I have always been a supporter of eating breakfast. Fortunately, I am one of those people who is pretty content eating the same meal over and over and over again, and breakfast is definitely a place where that tends to be my modus operandi. Mostly that's because I like it to be quick and predictable so I can speed up my getting-ready-for-the-day routine (especially on weekdays)! I tend to rotate between three different breakfasts (usually spending two to three months eating one before I switch to the other for two to three months, and then I'm back to the first). It's not exciting, but it works for me. You will need to find what works for you! Here are my breakfast of champion choices:

1. Oatmeal with ½ cup of blueberries and a handful of whatever nuts I have on hand-tossed in (walnuts, cashews, or almonds usually)

2. Greek yogurt with granola or nuts and a hard-boiled egg (I boil up a bunch of eggs at the beginning of the week, so they're ready to go when I need them!)

3. Two eggs scrambled with salt/pepper and eaten on a bed of spinach or with a slice of nut butter bread (which is a very simple "bread" consisting of 1 cup of any nut butter, three eggs, 1 tbsp. vinegar, 1 tsp. baking soda, and ½ tsp. of salt; bake at 350 degrees Fahrenheit for 25 minutes)

Getting Your Zs to Drop the LBs

Sleep is such a natural part of our life that we often don't think too much about it until we are going without it. I know I didn't give sleep that much thought until my daughter was born. The first few months of her life were the first real period of time that I went for long stretches without getting adequate amounts of sleep. Night after night, for months at a time, along with my wife, I slept for only short stretches at a time, which led to many changes in my body. I noticed a decrease in my ability to focus, changes in my normally calm and even personality, and even changes in my appetite.

Although for years prior, I had been inquiring about my patients' sleep patterns in order to help them lose weight, I had never personally experienced how sleep can impact satiety. However, now I can share from first-hand experience that changes in sleep can affect your appetite and your ability to feel satiated. Research backs up this lived experience as it shows that sleep is a key component to the regulation of the two hormones that influence hunger: leptin and ghrelin.

Leptin, along with peptide YY, is known as being the hormones that make you feel full, and ghrelin, as we know, is the hormone that makes you feel hungry. As previously discussed, the release of peptide YY is mainly influenced by food intake. This is also true in the case of leptin, which is usually at its lowest levels in the morning and slowly increases over the course of the day until it peaks at nighttime. Ghrelin is released by the stomach on a more incremental basis, quickly decreasing after a meal and increasing in anticipation of the next meal. These hormones work together to control satiety and hunger throughout the day. In addition to being affected by what type and how much food we eat, these hormones are also influenced by sleep.

During sleep, leptin levels rise, alerting your brain that you have plenty of energy (calories) on hand to get you through the night and that there's no need to trigger the feeling of hunger. However, when you don't get enough sleep, your body doesn't produce adequate amounts of leptin, and through a series of reactions, these low levels of leptin make your brain think that you don't have access to enough energy. As a result, you feel hungry, even though your body doesn't actually need food. This decrease in leptin brought on by sleep deprivation can result in persistent feelings of hunger, overeating, and a slow-down of your metabolism. Circulating ghrelin levels have also been found to be related to your sleep patterns.

As you are aware, the purpose of ghrelin is the opposite of leptin as it tells your brain when you need to eat, when it should stop burning calories, and when it should store energy as fat. During sleep, levels of ghrelin decrease because sleep requires far less energy than does being awake. However, if you don't sleep enough, then you end up with too much ghrelin in your system. This makes your body think that it's hungry, that it needs more calories, and as a result of these impulses, your body slows down your metabolism in order to conserve energy.

Both ghrelin and leptin are very connected to how much and how long you sleep. The Center for Disease Control recommends that adults sleep at least seven to nine hours per night. If you are meeting these sleep requirements, it is likely that your leptin and ghrelin levels are well balanced, but when sleep patterns are disrupted, ghrelin and leptin levels are disrupted as well.

This is true whether you miss out on getting enough sleep for as little as one day or chronically for weeks or months at a time. During a state of sleep deprivation, ghrelin levels rise, and leptin levels fall more than usual. This leads to a state in which you feel hungry even when your body does not need to eat. Research confirms that sleep deprivation leads to changes in circulating hormone levels, which can affect your eating behaviors.

A study conducted at the University of Wisconsin examined the relationship between sleep, leptin, and ghrelin levels, and BMI. After studying more than 1,000 volunteers, it was found that a dose relationship existed between sleep duration and body mass index. They discovered that habitual sleep duration of fewer than 7.7 hours a night was associated with significant changes in leptin and ghrelin and increased BMI[11]. These findings, which associate a lack of sufficient sleep with an increase in weight gain, were substantiated in a meta-analysis published out of King's College in London.

The meta-analysis combined the results of several research studies in an effort to determine if sleep deprivation leads to an increase in caloric consumption the following day. The results of the meta-analysis found that, on average, sleep-deprived people ate 385 extra calories per day. Interestingly, the analysis also showed that people who are sleep deprived are also more likely to eat a diet that is higher in fat and lower in protein[12]. As you might imagine, if, on average, you were to eat 385 extra calories the day after you were sleep-deprived, those who are chronically sleep-deprived would be much more likely to gain significant amounts of weight over time.

It's clear to see that sleep deprivation is linked to increased feelings of hunger, which have been shown to lead to weight gain. So if you are currently sleeping less than 7.5 hours a night, what can be done to help improve your sleep habits? The good news is that there are several lifestyle modifications that can be made in order to promote better sleep. Here are some options you might want to consider building into your weight loss plan:

Daytime Habits:

Exercise: Cardiovascular exercise increases the amount of slow-wave sleep, the deep sleep where the brain and the body have the chance to rejuvenate. This type of exercise can help to improve your mood and decrease feelings of depression and anxiety, which often hamper sleep. However, cardiovascular exercise can be stimulating, so it's usually best to perform exercise during the day or at least several hours before your target bedtime.

Reduce Stress: Chronic stress, as well as experiencing stressful events, can keep your brain active at night, making it challenging to sleep. In order to help your brain better prepare to "shut off" at night, you may consider practicing regular stress-reducing habits. These practices might include things like yoga, meditation, and deep breathing.

Exposure to Natural Light: Sunlight influences your body chemistry in order to keep you in sync with the natural progression of the day. By exposing yourself to sunlight first thing in the morning, you are altering your body to start its "circadian clock," which will, in turn, wind down as bedtime approaches. Eating breakfast near a window or taking a morning walk are ways in which you might consider gaining exposure to A.M. sunlight.

Eat a Healthy Diet: Eating a diet high in fiber and low in sugar and saturated fat throughout the day can help to promote better evening sleep. Research indicates that the more calories you consume from saturated fat and sugars, the more likely you are to wake up in the middle of the night[12]. This is most likely because sugar and fat interfere with the brain's production of serotonin, which you need for sleep.

Monitor Your Caffeine Intake: Caffeine is a stimulant that promotes alertness and keeps you from feeling sleepy. After caffeine is consumed, it takes many hours for your body to eliminate it from your system; as a result, if it is consumed in high doses or too close to bedtime, it can interfere with your ability to sleep. The American Academy of Sleep Medicine recommends limiting your caffeine consumption to no more than about 300-400 mg per day and avoiding caffeine consumption in the late afternoon and evening. Here are the caffeine levels found in a number of common products:

Product	Serving Size	Caffeine (mg)
Coffee	8 oz	95
Black Tea	1 C	55
Monster Energy Drink	16 oz	173
Diet Coke	12 oz	46.5

Evening Habits:

Avoid Eating Before Bed: Eating close to bedtime can lead to sleep disruptions, including taking longer to fall asleep, less time in REM sleep, and a greater likelihood of waking after falling asleep. These disruptions appear to be much more likely for people who consume high amounts of fats in the evening hours[13]. To improve your sleep quality, try to limit food consumption close to bedtime, and if you are going to eat after dinnertime, try to avoid high-fat foods.

Avoid Alcohol Consumption Before Bed: Alcohol helps to induce sleep, but it also makes your sleep more disrupted. This disturbance interferes with our REM sleep, which is the restorative part of sleep. To avoid these disruptions, try to limit how frequently you drink alcohol, and when drinking, try to finish your last drink at least three to four hours prior to your bedtime.

A Consistent Bedtime and Routine: Your body, just like everyone else's, loves routine. A consistent sleep schedule trains your brain to release hormones that induce sleep around the same time each night. Likewise, a regular bedtime routine gives your body and brain a chance to wind down in anticipation of sleep while helping signal the release of sleep-inducing hormones. To promote the consistent release of these hormones, try to keep your bedtime and routine consistent, seven days of the week. A consistent wake time will also help promote healthier sleep.

Shut Off Screens: Sleep disturbances related to screens are becoming a major concern in developed countries. The blue light given off from devices such as smartphones, tablets, computers, and televisions can suppress the release of sleep-inducing hormones. In order to ensure restful sleep, make your bedroom a "device-free space," manage your device settings so that your screens dim as bedtime approaches, and ideally, turn off all screens two to three hours before going to bed.

Make getting a full night of restful sleep a priority; it's certainly a habit that can lead to an increase in satiety, and that can promote weight loss. Sleep, along with how often we eat and what we choose to eat for breakfast, are important factors when it comes to how hungry we feel throughout the day. But what about when you decide to eat when you aren't feeling hungry? For a lot of people answering this question and creating behaviors to address their own answer to it is often the key to achieving significant and sustainable weight loss.

Katy: Sleep is hugely important for me, and is definitely something I have learned to prioritize in my life. It became even more important for me after I was diagnosed with an autoimmune disorder and I started to experience amplified effects of fatigue when I didn't get enough sleep. My ideal sleep target is seven to eight hours per night. I realize that may be difficult for some to achieve depending on individual life circumstances, but given the points Ryan has made, I hope you'll consider how you can improve your sleep habits and opportunities for good sleep.

Here are the reasons that I benefit from getting enough sleep:

- ✓ I am awake fewer hours of the day; thus, I have fewer hours in the day to be hungry!
- ✓ I can think more clearly when I have gotten enough sleep.

Here are the ways I have found to make sure I get enough sleep:

- ✓ Closing my kitchen by 8 p.m. means that my stomach is through the heavy periods of digestion by the time I'm heading to bed. I have learned that it is uncomfortable to go to bed when I've been eating, and my body is still processing food.

- ✓ Exercise and be active! When I tire my body out, sleep comes much more easily.

- ✓ I am prone to anxiety and stress. Doing things to calm my mind (prayer/meditation, reading a book before I fall asleep calms my mind and keeps my mind from spinning, listening to peaceful music) helps me fall asleep and stay asleep.

- ✓ Calculate what time I need to be up and going in the morning and work backward to give myself a target bedtime. For me, most of the time on weeknights, I am in bed by between 9:30-10 p.m. and up by 5:30–6 a.m. to exercise and then get ready for the day.

- ✓ I have learned I need to communicate with my family/friends that sleep is important to me. This sometimes means going to bed and/or heading home, even when things are still happening. In the beginning, this was hard! I felt like I was disappointing my family and friends, and I was also experiencing severe FOMO (fear of missing out) because I felt like a boring party pooper heading off to bed while the party was still happening.

✓ I am more emotionally stable when I am well-rested. When I have not slept enough, I am more prone to frustration, anger, and other mood swings. I just don't handle life as well.

✓ I don't have that overpowering urge for a nap in the afternoon.

✓ I have the energy I need to exercise, which is also good for my body!

✓ I am just simply a happier person (and I'm sure I'm much more pleasant to be around).

✓ I have learned to prioritize sleep. Now, I don't employ this tactic all the time, but sometimes I just need to call it and go to bed. I am so much happier the next morning when I do! Over time, my family and friends have come to respect my sleep needs and are supportive of my choices. That's what a healthy and helpful family and friends do!

Of course, there are times when I just simply don't get enough sleep. For you, that might happen in periods of times when there are significant family demands, job demands, or other life demands. When I have a stressful work deadline looming, I work longer days, and there are times that the nights get quite short because of late nights coupled with early mornings. When I am visiting my extended family, we tend to stay up late into the night talking, and the mornings come early so we can spend more time together. These situations are going to happen. When these times come (and there will always be times that they come!), I just have to roll with it and manage it. If they become chronic, I recommend looking for ways to adjust lifestyle choices and/or family schedules (or perhaps trading off family duties) to help you achieve whatever **your** ideal sleep goals are.

What's Next?

In the next chapter, we will take a deep dive into why we eat when we aren't hungry. By the end of this dive, you'll be able to decide if your weight-loss plan should include goals that help support making changes around emotional eating.

Chapter 6 Key Takeaways:

- The daily habits you practice can have a big impact on your ability to lose weight.

- Eating appropriately portioned-sized meals and snacks every three to four hours can help you avoid becoming overly hungry and overeating.

- Eating a high-protein breakfast has been shown to increase feelings of satiety and to promote weight loss.

- Aim to eat at least 15 grams of protein at breakfast each day.

- Sleep deprivation has been linked to increased appetite and weight gain.

- Sleeping at least 7.5 hours a night has been shown to increase feelings of satiety throughout the day.

Chapter 7

Emotional Eating

Having read the previous two chapters, I hereby deem you a practical expert on how to achieve physical satiety by making purposeful dietary and behavioral choices. As a result, I am fully confident that if your body alerts you that you are physically hungry, you'll know what to eat in order to satisfy this need while being able to stay within your caloric budget. However, responding to physical hunger is only half of the equation. The other half involves eating for reasons other than meeting your body's physical needs.

Eating to fill an emotional need rather than to satisfy physical hunger is most frequently referred to as emotional eating. Oftentimes food cravings generated by emotions are confused with physical hunger cues. The act of eating food in reaction to emotions such as boredom, happiness, loneliness, sadness, and joy is a part of many different cultures. When eating in reaction to these types of emotions is restricted to exceptional scenarios such as major life moments (good and bad), it is of little consequence to your weight or health. However, regularly eating to meet an emotional need rather than to fulfill physical hunger can make it challenging and oftentimes near impossible to lose weight. For this reason, it's important to learn how to recognize the difference between emotional and physical hunger.

Several psychosomatic theories regarding obesity suggest that people who are obese overeat due to their inability to perceive their physiological state, whether it be hunger or satiety. These theories also suggest that people who are obese often overeat to reduce feelings of emotional discomfort and anxiety[1,2,3]. Regardless of our BMI, most of us can recall a time when we turned to food to fill an emotional need rather than a physical need, such as eating a pint of ice-cream when you are feeling down after a bad breakup, eating numerous appetizers to calm your nerves during a social event where you don't know anyone, and eating sweets while you are watching TV home alone at night as an attempt to soothe the feeling of loneliness. The list of these scenarios could go on forever. If this type of eating only takes place in your life once in a blue moon, it's perfectly acceptable and will have little effect on your weight. But keep in mind that eating to fill an emotional need on a regular basis is a surefire way to sabotage your weight loss efforts. Emotional eating should be treated with particular importance by people living with a mood disorder such as anxiety or depression because, for them, the risk of chronically eating this way is much greater.

Mood Disorders and Emotional Eating

Anxiety and depression are frequently associated with chronic emotional eating. In fact, both anxiety and depression have been shown to be comorbidities of obesity[4,5,6]. Although anxiety and depression bring about very different feelings of psychological discomfort, eating to soothe these feelings of distress is a common response.

Anxiety

Anxiety, not to be confused with everyday stress, is categorized as an intense, excessive, and persistent worry and fear about everyday situations. Generalized anxiety disorder is one of the most prevalent mood disorders experienced by U.S. adults and can be felt on many different levels of intensity. The good news is that most often, anxiety can be well managed through lifestyle habits, counseling, and/or medication. However, often without realizing it, individuals dealing with chronic anxiety can fall into the habit of using food as a coping strategy. This co-occurrence of anxiety and overeating has been well researched.

Anxiety symptoms and disorders frequently co-occur with overeating, and studies have shown that those with Binge Eating Disorder have a greater likelihood of experiencing significant symptoms of anxiety compared with the general population[7]. Binge Eating Disorder is marked by regular episodes of eating an objectively large amount of food in a relatively short amount of time with a feeling of loss of control during the eating episode, with accompanying distress and impairment in one's life (i.e., health, social functioning, work performance). In one such study, anxiety was the most frequently cited among a list of emotions that trigger binge eating, followed by sadness, tiredness, anger, and happiness[8]. Thinking logically, this may not make much sense – what does food have to do with coping with anxiety? However, it has been shown that eating foods that trigger feelings of satisfaction within our brains, such as foods high in sugar and fat, can provide a feeling of instant, short-term relief for someone dealing with anxiety. This

141

instant feeling of relief may be one driving force for why people suffering from anxiety turn to food, but there are also other reasons that this might be true.

Some people coping with anxiety may look at food as an escape from self-awareness. The "escape" theory proposes that people looking to lose weight are particularly vulnerable to thinking about themselves in a negative way, which can result in feelings of anxiety[9]. To relieve themselves of these thoughts, they focus their attention on something that provides an immediate distraction, such as food. In addition to attempting to escape from their feelings by eating, some individuals with anxiety may try to use food as a way of regulating their emotions.

The term emotional regulation refers to a person's ability to identify and make sense of emotions while utilizing effective strategies for balancing these emotions[10]. Anxious people who struggle with emotional regulation will frequently look for methods of reducing their anxiety as quickly as possible, without giving much thought to the long-term ramifications. Foods that are high in fat and sugar can provide this immediate, albeit very short-term relief to ease these feelings of anxiety. Finally, people may look toward food to counteract their anxiety in the form of a "trade-off."

A trade-off does not help to reduce negative feelings but can be used to reduce the intensity of certain emotions[11]. That is to say, that anxiety could trigger someone to overeat because they dislike the way anxiety makes them feel, and they have learned that eating seems to make them feel better, at least temporarily. This person may know that they will feel a sense of guilt and even shame after overeating, but for them, the trade-off is acceptable because they at least get a short-term reprieve from the overwhelming feeling of their anxiety. Although generalized anxiety is the mood disorder most closely linked to emotional eating, people with depression have also been shown to be vulnerable to practicing chronic emotional eating.

Depression

Depression is a mood disorder that is characterized by a persistently depressed mood or loss of interest in activities, causing significant impairment in daily life. Depression is very common and very treatable. Similar to anxiety disorders, depression can be managed through lifestyle changes, therapy, and/or medication. However, if depression is left unaddressed or is not fully treated to remission, it can lead people to seek other short-term solutions to make themselves feel better, such as food.

People experiencing depression are more likely to consume foods that are high in fat and sugar in an attempt to relieve their negative feelings[58]. Although in the short-term, these types of foods can improve a person's mood, consistently eating foods that are high in fat and sugar can lead to weight gain[12,13,14].

It is easy to see that this pattern of eating foods that are high in fat and sugar in order to feel less depressed, temporarily feeling better, feeling down again, and eating more unhealthy foods to feel better can quickly turn into a vicious cycle that leaves an individual feeling unhappy and overweight. This cycle has been studied closely, and the research shows that over time, this repetitive eating of foods that contain high levels of fat and sugar leads to obesity[60].

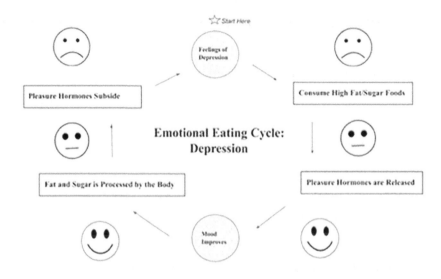

With the understanding that people who are dealing with anxiety and depression are more likely to practice emotional eating and that they are at greater risk for obesity, the question becomes, what, if anything, can be done about it? The answer is that for the most part, both feelings of anxiety and depression can be fully treated, and this treatment should take precedence over attempting to lose weight.

Diagnosis and Treatment of Mood Disorders

During my time at MGH, I worked with hundreds of patients with mood disorders who were also looking to lose weight. As you might imagine, I encouraged them to choose their own path towards weight loss: some decided to address their mood disorder upfront before attempting or while simultaneously trying to lose weight, while other patients firmly believed that losing weight would improve their mood and were adamant about attempting to lose weight before creating a plan to address their anxiety or depression. Inevitably, the patients who attempted to lose weight before addressing their mood disorder failed to achieve their weight-loss goal and wound up realizing that they needed to address their anxiety and/or depression before they would be able to have sustainable success losing weight. While on the other hand, plenty of my patients who decided to set goals that both supported their mental health needs and their weight- loss goal experienced great success. So although I, of course, encourage you to decide which path to weight loss is going to work best for you, if you have a mood disorder that is not currently treated to remission or believe that you might, I strongly recommend that you address this concern before attempting to lose weight.

Depending on the severity of your mood disorder, your symptoms can most often be managed through behavioral health approaches (exercise, planned joyful activities, mindfulness, etc.), counseling, and/or medication. If your depression or anxiety symptoms are moderate to severe, you may need to treat your symptoms by using several or all of these modalities. If your depression or anxiety is mild to moderate, just one of these interventions might be enough to achieve symptom remission. The best place to start the conversation around diagnosis and treatment is with your primary care physician. Together you can discuss your concerns, identify the severity of your symptoms, and create a treatment plan that will work best for you.

What If You Do Not Have a Mood Disorder but Are Still Struggling with Emotional Eating?

What if you are not someone who has a mood disorder but still finds yourself chronically eating in response to your emotions? If this describes you, there are steps that you can take to change your eating habits. These steps include recognizing the difference between physical and emotional hunger, pausing to understand why you are hungry, identifying your triggers, and substituting a way to address your emotions in place of food.

Recognizing Physical and Emotional Hunger

The first step in the process of curbing emotional eating is to start recognizing if your hunger is being driven by an actual physical need or in response to your emotions. Like any behavior that you are trying to change, this initial step is based on increasing self-awareness. In this case, increasing your self-awareness means improving your ability to recognize when you are feeling hungry because your body is looking for a source of energy and when your brain is telling you that it is hungry in order to address an emotional need. Let's take a look at some of the signs that you can begin to become aware of in order to tell the difference between physical and emotional hunger:

Signs of Physical Hunger	Signs of Emotional Hunger

Originates in the gut – manifests as a growling stomach or nausea	Originates in the brain – manifests as anticipation of how you will feel differently after you eat or as a fantasy about the taste of a particular food
Comes on gradually	Comes on suddenly
Can be satisfied with a variety of food options	Is met by eating a particular type of food
Signs of hunger will reside after nutritional needs are met	Your desire to eat may continue even after the point of feeling physically full and may result in feelings of guilt or shame after you eat

Now that you understand the signs that point towards physical or emotional hunger, if you find yourself looking to eat as a result of physical hunger, please use the knowledge you have already obtained about satiety in the last chapter to make a food choice that will satisfy your hunger while preserving the caloric deficit you are trying to achieve. On the other hand, if you determine that you are frequently feeling hungry as a result of emotional cravings, consider using the succeeding steps to change your eating patterns. This three-step process consists of pausing to identify the source of your hunger, identifying your triggers, and substituting a new behavior.

Pausing to Identify the Source of Your Hunger

Pausing to think about where your hunger is originating from is the hardest and the most critically important step towards changing a pattern of emotional eating. For most people that eat in response to their emotions, this reaction becomes an unconscious act. Therefore, in order to be able to disrupt the cycle of eating in reaction to your emotions, when you feel hungry, you must pause to ask yourself:

Am I Hungry Because of a Physical Need?

If Not, What Emotional Need Am I Trying to Meet?

Once you can get into the habit of pausing to recognize the source of your desire to eat, you can then take the next step, which is to identify what is triggering this drive to eat in the first place.

Identify Your Triggers

Identifying your food triggers starts by taking notice of the circumstances around you when you most often crave food. You can take notice of your environment by asking yourself the following questions:

1. ***What is happening around me right now?*** Did your boss just get upset with you? Did you just get off the phone with your judgmental mother? Are you home alone in the evening and looking for something to do?

2. ***What are you feeling inside?*** Are you feeling stressed, bored, or sad? Are you trying to soothe this uncomfortable feeling by eating?

The answers to these questions will help you to identify what type of situations/interactions typically trigger your desire to eat emotionally and pinpoint what type of emotion(s) you are trying to relieve with food. Once you have identified your triggers and the emotions you feel, you can then begin to use methods other than food to satisfy your emotional needs.

Substituting Other Behaviors in Place of Eating

An unsustainable way to address the concern of emotional eating would be to deny yourself the ability to meet your emotional needs through food without providing yourself with an effective substitute. In order to make the switch from soothing with food to another behavior, it is best to have an alternative behavior or action identified and ready to implement before your cravings hit. It is important to keep in mind that although your substitute behavior(s) will be unique, it should meet these two requirements:

1. *It is something you find pleasure in.*

2. *It will take your mind off of eating.*

As long as your substitute behavior meets these two criteria, it should be able to fill your emotional needs in place of food. Keep in mind that different emotions may require different substitute behaviors. That is to say that the actions that help to relieve your feelings of boredom may not help you feel better when you are stressed. Therefore, I would recommend that you come up with a variety of substitute behaviors so that you can apply them when and where they are most effective.

Advanced Coaching Tip: Create an Emotional Eating "Home Field Advantage"

It has been well documented that in sports, the team playing on their home field has a higher likelihood of winning. There are many factors involved in why the home team is more likely to win. One of these factors is that they are able to control the environment in order to tilt the odds of winning in their favor. You can create this same "home field advantage" where you live by creating an environment that minimizes the likelihood of emotional eating. Here are some tips on how to create a home environment that works to your advantage:

1. Food Shopping: If you are prone to emotional eating, it can be a great advantage to limit the amount of high fat/sugar foods that enter your home. Simply put: "if it isn't there, you can't eat it." To avoid bringing unhealthy foods home, make a list before you shop and try to stick to shopping the outer perimeter of the store where the produce and lean proteins are located, while only going down the center aisles you need to in order to pick up the items on your list.

2. Food Placement: Food manufacturers pay premium prices to have their products placed at the end of aisles and at eye level in grocery stores so that their items are more likely to be noticed and purchased. You can use this same strategy at home by placing foods that are higher in fat/sugar on very high or low shelves in your pantry or in the back of the refrigerator. Conversely, you can place healthier items at

150

eye level so that you are more likely to notice and consume those foods.

3. Accessible Alternatives: The substitute behavior(s) that you have come up with to replace eating in reaction to your emotions should be readily available within your home. For instance, if you plan to chew on gum rather than eating, make sure you have plenty of packs available and in eyesight. If your plan is to knit, have your knitting supplies stocked and ready to go somewhere in your living room. The easier you make it to access your food substitutes, the more likely you will be to use them.

Putting It All Together

Let's take the examples of eating in reaction to boredom and stress (two of the most common triggers of emotional eating) in order to illustrate what putting the four-step action plan of understanding the difference between physical and emotional hunger, pausing to recognize why you are hungry, identifying your triggers, and addressing your emotions without food looks like in action.

Boredom

Jon has just finished a long work week and decides to spend his Friday night relaxing at home. He is watching Netflix on the couch when he gets a sudden desire for an ice-cream sundae. He makes his way to the kitchen, but before opening the freezer, he *pauses* to *identify* where his desire to eat ice-cream is coming from. He notices that he is still feeling physically satiated from dinner, which he just finished forty-five minutes ago, that his hunger came on suddenly, and that his hunger is associated with a very specific food item. He recognizes that these signs point toward an emotional desire to eat rather than a physical need. Thinking about it more, he determines that this desire to eat has been *triggered* because he is bored. He is not really into this Netflix show, and he now wishes that he had gone out with his coworkers tonight. Since he has noticed in the past that he frequently eats as a result of boredom, Jon is prepared with a *substitute* behavior, which for him is playing video games online with friends. As a result, he decides to fire up his video-game system to see who is available to play and passes on the ice-cream sundae and the 600 calories that would have come with it.

Stress

Maryanne is having a typical day at work when her boss sticks his head into her office. He asks if she has completed the report that he wanted her to have finished by the end of the week. Since it is only Tuesday, she replies, "Not yet," which is retorted by her boss with, "You better have it to me by the end of the day." After her boss moves on, Maryanne reaches her hand into the candy bowl on her desk, which she leaves out for visitors. As she is about to unwrap her first piece of chocolate, she *pauses* to *identify* why she is eating it. She notices that she doesn't feel hungry because she just finished breakfast around an hour ago, her desire to eat the chocolate came on in an instant, and she only wanted something sweet to eat, which is why she has no desire to eat the apple in her bag. During this pause, she determines that she has been *triggered* by her boss to reach for the chocolate as an attempt to relieve her feeling of stress. Rather than eating the piece of chocolate and likely many more pieces after that, Maryann decides to go visit with her coworker Paula in order to *substitute* venting to a friend about her boss instead of eating.

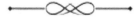

Katy: Emotional eating is a topic I have spent the past several years seeking to understand with greater clarity and intention because it is an area I have always struggled with. For as long as I can remember, highly emotional moments have been linked with some kind of food: Celebratory moments – "I finished Finals! It's my dog's birthday!"; devastatingly sad moments – "I didn't get the job I applied for. My best friend moved far away. That relationship didn't work out."; overwhelmed moments – "I'm in over my head at work. I don't even know where to start on this task,"; lonely moments – "I'm alone on a Friday night with no one to hang out with," etc. Within my personal culture, food has often been used as a medium to address emotions I am feeling and/or difficult experiences I am going through. There are the obvious links to emotional moments such as birthday or graduation celebrations, but then there are those that are not as readily apparent. As a kid, I played in a community softball league and, while I enjoyed playing in games, my favorite part of Game Day was waiting to see what treats were being provided afterward. But the snacks had little to do with sustenance and everything to do with the "reward" of playing the game.

There have been countless other ways I have been cultured to use food to address my emotions. Consider romantic comedies that suggest that the only way to handle a difficult breakup with a significant other is by drowning your sorrows in a pint of ice-cream or binge-eating a huge pile of junk food. Ironically, we have even been cultured to celebrate **health achievements** with food. Have you ever "rewarded" yourself with a food treat because you accomplished a physical feat such as going for a run (guilty), doing a hike (guilty), and/or because you took the stairs instead of the elevator (yes, guilty). I have spent the past several years trying to disentangle my physiological need for food from the psychological conditioning that food should be used as a reward/comfort/companion. This is **hard** to do. I'm still working on it. But, I am excited about the progress I've made and am hopeful that some things I've learned in the process will help you too.

How did I do it? Well, I'm a scientist, so naturally, I created a spreadsheet. I assure you, a spreadsheet isn't necessary; it's just something that worked for me. A few years ago, a lot piled up at one time. Professionally, I was very stressed about the next steps in my career and how I was going to manage an increasingly heavy workload in my new job. At the same time, I was dealing with some difficult personal health struggles that catapulted me into lots of emotional eating, for which I felt I had little control. I was eating food that wasn't good for me (because heaven knows that stress-eating doesn't involve me stuffing carrot sticks into my face) and was having difficulty stopping when I was full (why eat one cookie when I could go ahead and eat four!). What to do? I had done enough introspection to realize that my eating behaviors were connected to moments when I felt a lot of anxiety, and it was in those moments that I seemed to lose most of my rational thought around eating. So, I actually created a spreadsheet. If I found myself heading toward the kitchen/vending machine, I made myself stop and answer the questions in the spreadsheet. I asked myself questions about where I was (I wanted to understand whether certain settings were contributing to my urge to eat), what it was that I wanted to eat (was I looking for sweets, carbs, salty?), whether or not I was actually hungry at the moment (I wanted to know how often I was looking for food because I was **actually** hungry!), whether or not I was alone (I wanted to know whether it was easier/harder for me when I was with others or not), and whether or not I was feeling particularly anxious at that moment (because I suspected that anxiety was connected to my eating behaviors). My last question was always, "Did you follow through and eat?" and "How did you feel afterward about your decision to eat or not eat?" I learned a lot of things about myself with this exercise! I learned that most often, these urges to eat came when I was home and alone; I nearly always wanted something sweet, I rarely was actually hungry, and I often felt anxious in these moments. Doing this did two things for me. First, it made me stop at the moment to really consider whether or not I actually wanted to eat something. Just stopping to reflect interrupted the pattern of emotional eating for me and helped me to make a different decision. Many times, I chose not to eat anything at that moment because, by the time I finished answering the questions, I felt much more in control of my emotions than when I'd started. Secondly, I started to develop other coping strategies to deal with the difficult emotions and/or stress I was experiencing. If I felt the urge to eat, I'd go play the piano for a few minutes, go out for a quick walk, find someone to talk to, read a book for a little while, or just tell myself to get back to work!

Another aspect of emotional eating for me that has been difficult to navigate is the social-emotional contexts where food feels intertwined with my relationships. How many times have friends made goodies and generously dropped them off at my house to share? Students make treats to express gratitude for me helping them in some way. In these cases, I have such a hard time separating my appreciation for the kind gesture from my acceptance or refusal of the food itself. Somehow it feels like my refusal of the food is symbolically refusing the friendship, the kind gesture, and/or the person themselves. While I know in my head this doesn't make sense; the emotional part of me really struggles with it. Where did this notion come from? I come from a family where food itself is treated as a love language. Someone making or buying special food for you is equated as a particular token of love. I've done it myself too! Making food _feels_ like an expression of love.

After I moved out of my parents' house, I would specifically request certain meals when I came home for a visit because they tasted like home and family. My parents would lovingly make the food, and it was great. Truly great. In time, as my eating goals evolved, some of those foods became at odds with what I was willing to put in my body. The first time I attempted to refuse special food that had been made special for me upon my return home, I couldn't follow through. I felt like I had punched them in the gut, and I backed down and ate the food anyway. For several years, I decided I would just have to live with deviating from my eating plan/goals when I visited my family because I wanted to preserve the relationships more than I wanted to keep with my personal wellness vision. I had created a false dichotomy for myself: that I could either stick with my vision OR I could accept the love of my friends and family. I have since learned that I don't have to choose one or the other; I can do both! But how did I make that happen? Well, first, I had to be open with my family about what my personal vision for myself was. I had to actually communicate with them what I was working for and **why** the way I ate was so important to me. It was rather unfair of me to assume that my family was sabotaging my health goals when they had no idea why I had changed my eating behaviors. Remember, I had been eating the way I'd been eating for twenty-five plus years. How could they possibly have known I'd changed things up unless I told them? How could they help me if I didn't **tell** them what I wanted for my health?

I wish I could tell you that I communicated my health goals to my family and everything was peachy keen from there on out. Not so. When I began to be more vocal about my health goals and the things I wanted to eat (and/or not eat), my family was wonderful and began to adapt their expectations around what I was willing to eat. And that was really helpful. I started planning ahead for the things I was willing to eat (e.g., my mom's enchiladas, my dad's amazing caramel popcorn) and the other things that I would prepare to pass on. But, that doesn't mean there weren't hurt feelings and/or challenges along the way. I remember at one point my mom commenting that she was sorry that her way of preparing food didn't meet my standards anymore, but that she had always done her best. That was a hard moment. I have been (and will always be!) grateful for the sacrifice my parents made for me and my siblings' well-being growing up, including the delicious homemade food that they provided. I am not ungrateful for that at all. From her perspective, my mom saw my adopting a new eating lifestyle as a rejection of the eating lifestyle she had nurtured in me as a child; and, in turn, as a rejection of her. Ouch. That's not what I ever intended. Fortunately, after time passed, and we all got more used to how my eating habits had evolved, it became a nonissue.

My parents are now completely supportive of my wellness vision for myself, and I have tried to help them understand that I took the good I learned from them (my parents have always grown a large garden, so they taught me well how to prepare and eat a myriad of delicious veggies) and just added additional things I've learned along the way (I've taught them about making zucchini pizza and using spaghetti squash as a pasta substitute).

As I've made a concerted effort to improve my eating behaviors, specifically in the context of emotional eating, there are few handy hints I've learned that have helped me in this process. First, I have learned how important it is to plan and prepare for situations around food that I know are challenging for me. These situations include, but are not limited to: visiting family where food will often be used as an expression of love or celebration; particularly stressful times like the end of the semester or right before big deadlines at work; unanticipated social events where I have little control over the food offered; long days of traveling via air or car when I'm tired and have little control over the available food. Here are a few things I have learned to help mitigate the emotional challenges around eating in these situations:

1. When I'm visiting family or traveling, I try to anticipate foods I know I'll be encountering and decide ahead of time what I want to partake in and what I would prefer to pass on. For example, my family has a tradition of eating cinnamon rolls on Christmas morning. So far, I have always chosen to eat them without worrying about the consequence of whether they will push me over my calorie limit on that one day. It's a once/year treat, and they are very nostalgic for me. On the other hand, I am more willing to forego store-bought treats because I can eat them any old time if I want to, and I'd rather be eating the things that are truly special. Similarly, when traveling, I will choose to eat the foods that I am unable to get elsewhere (e.g., amazing pizza and gelato in Italy) and pass on the foods that I can get at home.

2. I log everything I eat. When things get very emotionally stressful, logging my food is one of the first things I start to slack on. In those instances where I **keep** logging, I always come out the other side so much better for it. So, my mantra is to log, log, log my food. The objectivity of

logging really helps me get the emotionality of eating under better control.

3. I maintain my policy of no snacking late at night even when traveling. At my house, my kitchen is "closed" after 8:00 p.m. When I'm traveling or when I'm with my family, I try to abide by the same policies. Now, there are occasional exceptions but overall, I have learned that it is easier to sustain my wellness vision if I avoid late-night snacking.

4. I always carry gum. Sometimes my mouth just thinks it wants to chew something. I have learned to always have gum on hand so that I can pop a piece in my mouth and satisfy that craving without consuming food that, in the end, I don't really want.

5. When I'm in a particularly stressful/emotional moment, I no longer fill out a spreadsheet, but I do verbally ask myself the same kinds of questions: "Katy, why are you looking for food to eat? Are you really hungry? What is making you anxious right now? Is there something else you could be doing instead?" This kind of verbal reasoning with myself really helps manage my emotional impulse to eat.

6. Lastly, I have learned that sometimes the best strategy is to limit my access to foods that are difficult for me to resist. I have a number of foods on the "no-can-buy" list because I have learned that if I have easy access to them, it is very challenging for me to avoid them. You might

have some of these too. For me, these include sweet treats, empty calorie snacks like chips, cookies, or pretzels, and even ice-cream. Now, importantly, I don't tell myself I can't have these foods. I just make it harder to get access to them! I have a rule for myself to not have any cartons of ice-cream in my freezer. If I want ice-cream, I need to go and buy some at the local ice-cream shop. I give myself permission to go whenever I want to go, but I just have to go and get it as opposed to having it readily available in my own freezer. This system works well for me. I have learned if I have to work a little harder to get the food the emotional part of me is saying it wants, I'm more able to control the outcome.

Mastering the challenges surrounding emotional eating has been (and continues to be) one of the biggest hurdles in maintaining my health. Sometimes I have big wins (like the time I prepackaged every snack in preparation for a work trip and didn't once buy food at the airport), and then other times I fall hard (like the time I ate the whole plate of cookies a friend had given me as condolences just on the car ride home. As in, the cookies didn't even make it in the house!). Thankfully, over time, the wins are coming with a higher degree of frequency, and the falls are getting to be fewer and farther in between. In all of this, I have taken to heart the mantra that stumbling emotionally is just that: a stumble. One of the best things I have learned is that every day is a new day. It's such a cliche, but it's absolutely true. A tough day of emotional eating does not have to automatically become a tough week/month/year of eating. There have been so many times I've gotten to the end of the day and reflected that it just didn't go well at all. And I've learned to remind myself that a new day will dawn and I can try again. That attitude has helped me immensely. Because life is life, I know that I will continue to have days and moments that will be challenging emotionally – but I am ever confident that I will get better at managing my eating, despite the inevitable emotional ups and downs of life. I am continually seeking ways to improve my habits, set myself up for success in emotional moments, and in time, I will continue to add to my arsenal of strategies so that my food habits aren't dictated by what's happening emotionally in my life.

What's Next?

In addition to using this four-step method to change your emotional eating habits, it is important to note that creating lifestyle habits that include a balance of exercise, healthy eating, and sleep will certainly reduce your emotional cravings to eat. Building these types of lifestyle habits in combination with using the recognize, pause, identify, and substitute method should provide you with the tools you need to reduce the frequency in which you find yourself emotionally eating. One of these lifestyle habits that has been shown to improve your mood and support sustained weight loss is performing cardiovascular exercise, which will be the focus of the next chapter.

Chapter 7 Key Takeaways:

- Emotional eating has been linked to excess weight gain.

- People who have anxiety and/or depression are more likely to experience emotional eating.

- Treating anxiety and depression symptoms to remission will improve weight-loss results.

- Emotional eating can be reduced by practicing the recognize, pause, identify, and substitute method.

Chapter 8

Cardiovascular Exercise

Over the years, the idea of what type of exercise you need to perform in order to lose weight has been sensationalized and has often been taken to an extreme. Thanks to ideas portrayed on television and social media, there are many people who believe in the misconception that in order to lose weight, they need to be flipping giant tires, swinging heavy ropes, and pouring thousands of dollars into the hands of a personal trainer. Of course, this is entirely untrue. Although almost all successful and sustainable weight loss plans include regular cardiovascular exercise; you are not required to hire a personal trainer or to exercise in a warehouse or an airplane hanger in order to lose weight. In fact, I would encourage most people to take a completely different approach.

Before we get into all of the ways in which cardiovascular exercise helps to promote weight loss and what approach might work best for you, let's take a moment to understand what this term means. Cardiovascular exercise is any type of intentional, planned, and repetitive movement that raises your heart rate above its resting rate for an extended period of time. In order to understand how to design a cardiovascular exercise routine that will promote weight loss, we must return to the concept of creating a caloric deficit.

Creating a Caloric Deficit Through Cardiovascular Exercise

As we discussed previously, creating a caloric deficit is what leads to weight loss. A caloric deficit is predominantly created through eating fewer calories than you normally would; however, performing cardiovascular exercise can help add to the creation of a caloric deficit by helping you burn extra calories, increasing your metabolism, suppressing your appetite, and enhancing your mood.

Burning Extra Calories

The most well-known way that cardiovascular exercise aids in the creation of a caloric deficit is by causing your body to burn extra calories through repetitive movement. As you may recall, there are 3,500 calories in 1pound of fat; thus, in order to lose 1pound, you must create a caloric deficit of 3,500 calories. Over the course of a week, this would equate to the creation of a caloric deficit of 500 calories per day. For most of us, it is unrealistic and unsustainable to burn 500 extra calories a day by performing cardiovascular exercise. However, it is very realistic to use regular cardiovascular exercise to aid in the creation of a caloric deficit when used in combination with a dietary caloric reduction. In fact, enhancing weight loss through regular cardiovascular exercise is an area that has been well studied.

One such study, which was published in *Obesity,* examined how cardiovascular exercise affected 141 obese or overweight people over a ten-month period. Study participants were instructed not to reduce their dietary calorie intake and were then split into three groups:

165

Group 1: Burn 400 calories by performing cardiovascular exercise, five days a week

Group 2: Burn 600 calories by performing cardiovascular exercise, five days a week

Group 3: No exercise

Group 1 participants lost an average of 4.3 percent of their body weight, while those in group 2 lost a little more at 5.7 percent of their initial body weight. Group 3, which did not exercise, actually gained 0.5 percent more than their initial body weight[1]. Other studies support similar findings as they have shown that cardiovascular exercise can help you burn fat, especially abdominal fat, which has been shown to increase your risk of type 2 diabetes and heart disease[2,3,4]. In order to put this research into actionable terms, let's examine an example of what this might look like in a real-life setting.

For this example, let's consider Melissa, who has built a weight-loss plan that involves losing one pound per week by reducing her caloric intake by 500 calories per day. In order to enhance her results, Melissa decides to start taking a brisk, thirty-minute walk, five days a week, during her lunch break. During these walks, she burns 200 calories. By burning an extra 1,000 calories (200 calories, five days a week) per week, her total caloric deficit increases to 4,500 calories per week. Over the course of a year, this addition of a thirty-minute walk, five days a week, will help Melissa lose an extra 15 pounds (1000 calories x 52 weeks = 52,000 calories/ 3,500 calories = 14.86 pounds).

As you can see, the inclusion of even a moderate yet consistent amount of cardiovascular exercise can make a big difference when it comes to weight loss. In addition to increasing your caloric deficit through burning extra calories, cardiovascular exercise can also enhance caloric deficit creation by increasing your metabolism.

Increase in Metabolism

As we just discussed, one way in which cardiovascular exercise can help you to create a caloric deficit is by burning calories while you are exercising. However, in addition to the calories burned while you're working up a sweat, cardiovascular exercise has an additional benefit: it can help increase your metabolism through a post-cardiovascular exercise effect called the "afterburn."

The afterburn effect is formally known as EPOC, which stands for excess post-exercise oxygen consumption. After working out, your body needs to take in oxygen at a higher rate than it did pre-exercise so that it can cool down and repair itself. This restoration process requires your metabolism to work at a higher rate, during which it will continue to burn extra calories. The exact amount of calories burned will vary for each person, but research shows that EPOC can increase calorie burn by 6 to 15 percent[5,6]. The amount of calories you burn during EPOC is dependent upon the type of workout you just completed.

The longer and more intensely you exercise, the more time your body will spend in EPOC after you complete your workout. This makes sense because your body will have to spend more time cooling itself down and repairing cells if you have worked out for a long period of time and/or at a high intensity. Depending on the length and intensity of your workout, your body could continue burning calories at this increased rate anywhere from a few hours to well beyond 24 hours after exercise.

The additional calories burned during EPOC can help to boost your weight loss by aiding in the creation of a caloric deficit. On top of burning calories during exercise and EPOC, performing a cardiovascular exercise can also contribute to the creation of a caloric deficit by suppressing your appetite.

Appetite Suppression

What a magical beast cardiovascular exercise is, as it can help you burn extra calories, increase your metabolic rate, and make you feel less hungry. That's basically the weight loss trifecta! Appetite suppression after you workout is made possible by the effect that cardiovascular exercise has on your hormones.

Performing cardiovascular exercise has been shown to suppress ghrelin, that same hormone that we discussed earlier, which increases appetite. Exercising has also been shown to increase levels of peptide YY, which, as you know, is a hormone that suppresses appetite[7]. Sounds like a win, win, right? Yes, a total win, but you have to make sure you exercise long enough for appetite suppression to take effect.

Like EPOC, the level in which your appetite will be suppressed after you finish your cardio workout is dependent on how long you exercise for, how intense your exercise session is, and what type of cardiovascular exercise you perform. According to the American Physiological Society, appetite suppression will kick in after you have performed about sixty minutes of cardiovascular exercise. But the intensity in which you exercise also contributes to the level at which your appetite is suppressed.

Exercising more rigorously will reduce your appetite to greater levels than exercising moderately or gently, although moderate and light exercise has also been shown to help suppress appetite[8]. However, if you are looking to maximize post-exercise appetite suppression, it is best to exercise vigorously, as appetite has been shown to be suppressed for up to twenty-four hours after exercising, particularly for individuals who exercise strenuously[8]. In addition to working out at a strenuous level, you should also consider the mode of cardiovascular exercise you are performing in order to maximize appetite suppression.

Weight-bearing exercises have been shown to be more likely to result in suppressed appetite compared to non-weight-bearing exercises. Therefore, you may want to consider cardiovascular activities such as running or using the elliptical instead of biking or swimming if your goal is appetite suppression. Although cardiovascular exercise, if implemented with intent, can help to reduce your appetite by adjusting your hormone levels, it can also help you achieve the caloric deficit you are aiming for by improving your mood.

Mood Enhancement

What we end up calling our "diet" is really just a sum total of the food we eat, which is derived from the numerous decisions we make regarding food each day. We make hundreds of decisions every day, and many of them involve choices related to food intake, like what to eat, how much to eat, when to eat, and how often to eat. As humans, we make our most sound decisions when we are of a clear and healthy mind; however, when we are feeling down, anxious, or rushed, it is easy for us to make regrettable choices. Therefore, if your goal is to make food decisions that, when compounded, result in the creation of a caloric deficit, it is best to make these decisions when you are feeling mentally well. Cardiovascular exercise can help aid in this process by enhancing your mood, which leads to fewer incidents of emotional eating and an increase in how often you make healthy food decisions.

The psychological effects of cardiovascular exercise cannot be overlooked when it comes to weight loss. When you perform cardiovascular exercise, your body is stimulated to release dopamine, norepinephrine, and serotonin. These brain chemicals play an important role in regulating your mood. An enhanced mood can help you feel more at ease with yourself, which can facilitate a decrease in emotional eating and increase the rate of healthy decision-making, especially if you are dealing with high levels of stress or a mood disorder such as depression and/or anxiety.

Performing cardiovascular exercise can also serve as an interruption to the flow of constant worries running through your head. When we are feeling stressed and anxious, we are more likely to make food decisions based on our emotions, which are often irrational. However, when we are relaxed, we are more likely to make food choices based on physical needs, which supports the creation of a caloric deficit. In addition to reducing our feelings of stress and anxiety, cardiovascular exercise can improve our mood and reduce feelings of depression.

As mentioned earlier, feelings of depression can lead an individual to use the consumption of "comfort foods" as a form of relief. In addition to counseling and medication, exercise has been shown to help treat depressive symptoms. In fact, studies show that exercise can treat mild to moderate depression as effectively as antidepressant medication but without the side effects. As one example, a study conducted by the Harvard T. H. Chan School of Public Health found that running for fifteen minutes or walking for sixty minutes a day reduces the risk of major depression by 26 percent[9]. Exercise is a powerful depression fighter for several reasons. Most importantly, it leads to all kinds of changes in the brain that promote feelings of calm and well-being. In addition to releasing dopamine, norepinephrine, and serotonin that energize your spirits and make you feel good, exercise can also serve as a distraction. For individuals with depression, exercise can allow for some quiet time for their mind, which allows them to break out of the cycle of negative thoughts that feed depression.

So now you know that exercise supports weight loss through the creation of a caloric deficit by helping you burn extra calories, increasing your metabolism, suppressing your appetite, and enhancing your mood. At this point, you might be wondering how do I design a cardiovascular exercise routine that will support these mechanisms in order to lose weight? To design such a plan, you must consider cardiovascular exercise duration, mode, and intensity.

Duration, Mode, and Intensity

At this point, you should have a good understanding of how cardiovascular exercise can help you to achieve a caloric deficit. What I don't yet expect you to understand is how vigorously, how long, how often, and what type of cardiovascular exercise you should be performing in order to lose weight. However, by the end of this section, you'll have this down pat from learning the exercise guidelines that have been put together by the American College of Sports Medicine.

Cardiovascular Exercise Intensity

The levels of cardiovascular exercise intensity that have been shown to promote weight loss are lumped into two categories: moderate and vigorous. You are considered to be working out at a level of moderate exercise intensity when you are exercising at a heart rate of at least 40 percent of your maximum heart rate. In more tangible terms, this means that you are moving at a pace that is slow enough that it allows you to carry on a conversation but fast enough so that you aren't able to sing or whistle. The most common forms of moderate cardiovascular exercise are walking and cycling. Exercising at vigorous intensity is achieved when you are working out at a heart rate of at least 60 percent of your maximum heart rate. This can also be defined by exercising strenuously enough to the point where you are unable to carry on a conversation, and you are working up a sweat. The target duration and frequency of your exercise routine will depend on whether you are working at a moderate or vigorous intensity.

Cardiovascular Exercise Duration and Frequency

Of course, we all know that a relationship exists between how long you perform cardiovascular exercise and the amount of weight you'll lose. Clearly, the longer your exercise bout, the more calories you'll burn, and the longer you will be in EPOC, which helps you create a caloric deficit. With that said, I'd like to pass on some minimal exercise duration goals that, if met, will help you to lose weight and will lead to additional health benefits (lower blood pressure, cholesterol, blood sugars, the risk for certain types of cancers, etc.). If you are exercising at a moderate pace, you should aim for at least 150 minutes of exercise each week (i.e., 30 minutes x 5 a week). If you are exercising at a vigorous pace, your goal should be to exercise for at least 60 minutes a week (i.e., 20 minutes x 3 days a week). Or some combination of the two.

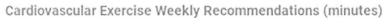

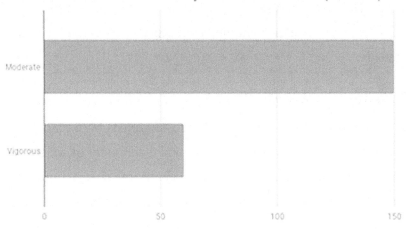
Cardiovascular Exercise Weekly Recommendations (minutes)

Cardiovascular Exercise Mode

The last factor to consider when developing a cardiovascular exercise routine is the mode or what type of exercise you'll be performing. As we'll get into later in this section, you'll read about how the "best" mode of cardiovascular exercise is one that you'll enjoy. With that said, here are a few of the most common types of cardiovascular exercise people often perform:

Moderate	Vigorous
Walking	Running
Moderate Cycling	Elliptical
Water Aerobics	Aerobic group exercise classes/videos
Hiking	Rowing

Creating a Sustainable Cardiovascular Exercise Routine

You've learned about how integrating regular cardiovascular exercise into your weekly routine can promote weight loss by helping you create a caloric deficit, and hopefully, you understand the guidelines that should be used for creating an exercise routine. Now it is time to consider how you might build a sustainable cardiovascular exercise routine into your life. Knowing the guidelines is one thing but actually putting them into practice is a completely different story. In order to make sure that you are successful with this part, if you choose to make performing regular cardiovascular exercise part of your weight loss plan, I would encourage you to consider four important factors: convenience, enjoyment, flexibility, and prioritization.

Putting It All Together

Cardiovascular exercise, when implemented in a sustainable way, can be of great benefit to anyone who has a goal of losing weight. An effective cardiovascular exercise routine should meet the following criteria:

1. It is fun

2. It is convenient

3. It is flexible

4. It is scheduled as a priority

It should also follow these American College of Sports Medicine guidelines:

1. If exercising at a moderate intensity, you should aim for a minimum of at least 150 minutes per week

2. If exercising at a vigorous intensity, you should aim for a minimum of at least 60 minutes per week

3. Or some combination of the two

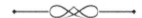

Katy: If I could distill down to one piece of advice the key to my own success for integrating cardiovascular exercise, it would be this: Start where you are. When I first began incorporating cardiovascular exercise into my life, the walks I was taking could hardly be described as cardiovascular or exercise. I wasn't breaking a sweat, I wasn't out of breath, nor was I speedily passing anyone on the path as I walked. I was merely getting out and taking a leisurely stroll around the block after dinner or driving down to the bike path along the river after work to go for a short (and I mean, very short) walk down the trail. My concept of cardiovascular exercise at that time included things like running a marathon, sweating it out in zumba, and/or riding in spin classes, which felt overwhelming and impossible for me to do. I was just not physically or mentally capable of that kind of exercise. And I believe **that's okay**. The reality was, starting off with easy walks was exactly where I needed to **start** on my path to incorporating an appropriate level of cardiovascular exercise into my life.

As Ryan has explained, cardiovascular exercise is any type of intentional, planned, and repetitive movement that raises your heart rate above its resting rate for an extended period of time. Using that definition, my little walks did technically count as cardiovascular exercise simply because it was more physical activity, albeit minimally so, than I was used to. But it didn't **feel** like cardiovascular exercise to me because I wasn't wearing workout clothes and/or sweating profusely. Even so, this was exactly the kind of exercise my body was physically capable of at the time. My lifestyle was primarily sedentary at that point. I was used to spending the day sitting at work, sitting in my car to and from work, and sitting on my couch at home in the evenings. Climbing a flight of stairs left me out of breath. I looked for parking spots that required minimal walking. I disliked walking between buildings at school or work because it didn't take much for me to work up a sweat and ruin my hair. So, in reality, small, short walks were the perfect place to start to build up my physical strength.

In order to successfully start where I was, I had to ignore what others said about what "counted" as cardiovascular exercise and listen to my own body. Starting where you are affords you the opportunity to build a routine of exercise (whatever that exercise looks like for **you**) without exhausting or overwhelming yourself. For me, starting where I was meant that I went for a short walk every day after work. I didn't put any constraints on how long the walk needed to be nor did I dictate any speed or intensity. I just decided to go for a walk every day. Was it hard for me to go on those walks? It was! The physical challenge, while there, was only part of the difficulty. The hardest part was remembering to go and do it! I was used to heading straight home after work to snack and eat dinner, watch a movie, and chill out on the couch. Going for a walk meant that I was going to have to disrupt that routine in some way and that was hard for me! Because I had permission to count a walk of any distance or any intensity as my walk for the day, it made it easier to build it into a habit.

As I built up the number of days I consecutively went for a walk, I began to feel successful with the exercise I was doing. If I had had the mindset right off the bat that the only exercise that "counted" was strenuous exercise beyond my current capabilities, I very likely would have become discouraged rather quickly. What I've learned over time is that by starting where you are, not only are you more likely to maintain your routine because the task does not feel impossible, you slowly **build** on what your body can physically do. When I started, I was able to walk only short distances comfortably. After a few weeks, I felt like I could start walking a little bit further. And then a little bit further. Eventually, I was consistently walking a couple of miles on every walk. And I was **proud** of that! I knew how hard it had been for me to go for a walk every day and I knew how hard I'd had to work to build up to walking two miles comfortably. It didn't matter to me what the world's standard of cardiovascular exercise was, I was proud of the change I could already see in my own life. Climbing one flight of stairs didn't phase me anymore (climbing two flights still left me out of breath). That was progress I could see as a result of a cardiovascular change happening in my own body!

"Start where you are" **for me** meant I started with going for a walk every day after work. As you consider where **you** are, you might choose to start with something else. Maybe walking isn't a challenge for you right now, so maybe your version of "start where you are" is working toward running a 5K. Maybe your "start where you are" is that you choose to take the stairs instead of taking the elevator at work. Maybe your version of "start where you are" is riding a bike around the block every day. Or, maybe it's doing a short workout routine from a YouTube video. It doesn't matter what **anyone else's** "start where you are" is; **you** know **your** body and **you** know what represents a physical challenge to **you**. When you start where you are, you figure out what your body is capable of and then you can start building on that. After I had been going for walks every day after work for several months (and was consistently walking three miles at a time), I recognized I needed and wanted a change in physical demands. So I started getting up before work and walking <u>before</u> work. Little by little, I started finding other ways to engage in other forms of cardiovascular exercise. I learned that I really enjoyed kayaking, biking, and hiking and that these were great forms of exercise for my body and my lifestyle. I learned that exercise classes such as zumba and spin classes weren't really my cup of tea. It's important to figure out what works for **you**. When you enjoy the exercise you're doing, you're much more likely to **continue** exercising.

At this point, cardiovascular exercise is one of the things I most rely on to center me and keep me grounded on my continued health journey. It has been a constant in my life for the past several years, and my day just doesn't feel complete anymore without some kind of physical activity. I like to do my exercise first thing in the morning. I try to mix things up so I don't get bored with what I'm doing. Sometimes I'll go for a jog in the neighborhood outside (when the weather is nice), or a hike on a local trail, or sometimes I'll go to the gym and take a turn on the elliptical, treadmill, or stair stepper.

I'd like to add one final thought to what has helped me be successful in maintaining a consistent routine of cardiovascular exercise. I am a strong believer in the importance of sound equipment that works well and is of high quality. This includes shoes. I have decided to make it a priority to make sure my shoes are of good quality and providing the appropriate support for my ankles, knees, and back. It's strange, I know, but I have learned that when my lower back starts to hurt, it's almost guaranteed that my shoes have worn down. A few years into my exercise routine, I splurged and bought a good quality bike that again, turned out to be a game changer. I spent hours on that bike putting in literally hundreds of miles over the course of several years. Later I added a road bike to my collection to give me more cycling options. It has been eye-opening and **fun** to acquire new hobbies and skills along my journey of incorporating steady, consistent exercise into my life. The key to this has been finding activities that I enjoy, setting little challenges for myself, and occasionally changing things up so I don't get overworked or bored with one activity.

What's Next?

If you implement a cardiovascular exercise routine based on the recommendations made in this chapter, then it should prove to be effective and sustainable. In addition to considering making regular cardiovascular exercise part of your weight-loss plan, I'd also recommend giving some thought to making strength training part of your plan, which is the topic we'll cover in the next chapter.

Chapter Eight Key Takeaways:

- Cardiovascular exercise helps you create a caloric deficit by allowing you to burn extra calories, by increasing your metabolism, by suppressing your appetite, and enhancing your mood.

- The American College of Sports Medicine recommends that you perform 150 minutes of moderate-intensity cardiovascular exercise or 60 minutes of vigorous cardiovascular exercise each week.

- Sustainable cardiovascular exercise routines are enjoyable, convenient, flexible, and prioritized.

Chapter 9

Strength Training

If I were to guess, I'd estimate that at least 40 percent of you considered skipping this chapter. I get it; you are interested in losing weight, not packing on muscle to become some sort of bodybuilder. But the truth is that 95 percent of people, myself included, do not have the genetic makeup to build muscle from strength training in a way that would allow them to look like a professional wrestler or to start winning bodybuilding competitions, even if they wanted to. Luckily, you don't need to add this type of muscle mass in order to gain the benefits from strength training that lead to sustained fat loss.

If I were to ask a room full of people what type of exercise helps to promote weight loss, I'd probably receive answers like running, biking, swimming, dancing, aerobics, playing team sports, and about twenty other ideas before someone would mention strength training. These answers certainly wouldn't be wrong; as we just discussed in the last chapter, there is no doubt that performing cardiovascular exercise aids weight-loss efforts but believe it or not, performing strength training is actually a stronger weight-loss catalyst.

You absolutely burn many more calories during cardiovascular exercise when compared to strength training; in fact, you burn very few calories when you are performing the act of strength training. However, when instituted on a regular basis, strength training has a much larger effect on your resting metabolic rate, which greatly influences fat loss, even when you are at rest. In this chapter, you will learn about the effect that strength training has on your resting metabolic rate, how strength training can help you preserve muscle while losing fat, and how to design a strength-training routine that will lead to significant weight loss.

Boosting Your Metabolism Through Strength Training

Have you ever heard someone say, "Oh, they're just thin because they have a fast metabolism"? There is some truth in this statement, as your metabolic rate certainly influences your weight. However, what I don't appreciate about this statement is that it implies that someone is thin solely due to their metabolic rate and excludes the healthy decisions they are probably making on a daily basis in order to maintain a healthy weight. It also implies that they have been given a fast metabolism when, in fact, up to 80 percent of someone's metabolic rate can be influenced by their behaviors.

Your resting metabolic rate is the amount of energy required to maintain your body's essential functions when it is at a resting state, such as respiration, blood circulation, gastrointestinal functions, and renal processing. Resting metabolic rate is the largest contributor to your body's total energy expenditure, accounting for approximately 65 to 70 percent of daily caloric burn[1,2,3]. Your resting metabolic rate is influenced by three factors: age, genetics, and body composition. Clearly, the first two factors are out of your control; however, your body composition is something you can manipulate to your advantage in order to enhance your weight loss results.

Body composition is considered your body's ratio of fat to lean body mass. As you may recall, even at rest, a muscle cell is metabolically much more active than a fat cell. As a result, variations in the ratio of fat to lean body mass account for approximately 70 to 80 percent of the difference in resting metabolic rate among individuals[4,5,6].

Strength training is the most effective way to add muscle tissue, and therefore it is also the best way to increase your resting metabolic rate. Strength training is any exercise that causes your muscles to contract against an external resistance with an expectation of increasing strength. The external resistance can be generated by using free weights, plated weight-lifting machines, exercise tubing, or your own body weight. When you perform strength-training exercises, microscopic tears are created in your muscle cells, which are quickly repaired by your body in order to help the muscles regenerate and grow stronger. When performed regularly, this cycle of muscle breakdown, repair, and growth, is what leads to an increase in muscle tissue and an increase in resting metabolic rate. Research has shown that when performed regularly, strength training can increase your resting metabolic rate by as much as 7 percent[7,8].

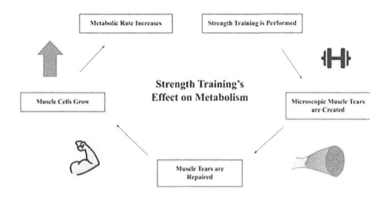

Strength Training's
Effect on Metabolism

Metabolic Rate Increases

Strength Training is Performed

Muscle Cells Grow

Microscopic Muscle Tears are Created

Muscle Tears are Repaired

An increase in your resting metabolic rate through the creation of muscle cells results in your body burning more calories while at rest. This means that when you're driving, sitting at your desk, and even sleeping, you'll be burning extra calories[9,10]. When looked at over the course of a period of months or years, this equates to a great deal of weight loss. In fact, several studies have shown that approximately 4 pounds of fat loss have been reported when people participate in ten weeks of a strength training program[11]. Extrapolated out conservatively over the course of a year, this means that there is a potential for upwards of 15-20 pounds of fat loss from incorporating regular strength training into your weekly routine. Still not sold that strength training can help to promote weight loss? Let's consider what happens to your resting metabolic rate if you decide to lose weight through caloric restriction without incorporating strength training into your routine.

Weight Loss in the Absence of Strength Training = Muscle Loss

As you know, creating a caloric deficit is essential to losing weight. When your body senses that it is experiencing a caloric deficit, it begins searching for sources of energy other than food. This is a good thing, as it will begin to use stored fat cells for energy. However, it will also begin to break down muscle tissue for energy as well[12]. In fact, it's been estimated that when people lose weight through caloric restriction, about a quarter of the weight loss is actually muscle tissue[13]. In the short term, this might not bother you – hey, you are losing weight, who cares what type of tissue it is? Right, except in the long-term, this loss of muscle tissue will result in a decrease in your metabolic rate, making it harder for you to keep losing weight and to avoid gaining it back.

A recent study showed that a typical person would experience a loss of 0.45 pounds of muscle mass and 0.55 pounds of fat mass for each pound of weight lost while dieting, without exercise[13]. Let's take a look at how this might play out when observed over time through a case study.

Emily has made many recent improvements to her diet and has been tracking her calories on a daily basis. As a result, she has been creating a daily caloric deficit of 500 calories per day and, as a result, has been losing 1 pound each week. However, she hasn't been performing strength training, so her weight loss has been a result of losing a mix of fat and muscle tissue. Here's what her fat/muscle loss ratios look like after five weeks of dieting:

Weight (lbs)	Fat Loss (lbs)	Muscle Loss (lbs)
200	0	0
199	.55	.45
198	1.1	.9
197	1.65	1.35
196	2.2	1.8
195	2.75	2.25

As you can see in the process of losing 5 pounds, solely through caloric restriction, Emily has only lost 2.75 pounds of fat while the other 2.25 pounds of her weight loss are attributed to the loss of muscle tissue. Therefore, Emily hasn't greatly altered her fat to muscle ratio, which means her resting metabolic rate has barely improved.

Now let's play out the same 5 pounds of weight loss as if Emily had been performing strength training in addition to restricting her calories. This is what her progress would look like:

Weight (lbs)	Fat Loss (lbs)	Muscle Loss (lbs)
200	0	0
199	1	0
198	2	0
197	3	0
196	4	0
195	5	0

In this scenario, Emily has lost 5 pounds of fat from caloric restriction, and she has maintained her muscle tissue by performing regular strength training. As a result, her fat to muscle ratio has shifted significantly, which will positively impact her resting metabolic rate, leading to the acceleration of further weight loss.

Weight loss research confirms that performing strength training in combination with caloric restriction leads to fat loss and the maintenance of muscle tissue and one's resting metabolic rate. In fact, a study that observed forty-eight overweight women eating a very-low-calorie diet found that those who followed a strength training program maintained their muscle mass, metabolic rate, and strength, even though they lost weight[14]. The women in the study who didn't perform strength training lost weight too, but they also lost more muscle mass and experienced a drop in their metabolic rate.

To summarize, if you restrict your calories in order to lose weight, without performing strength training, you will lose weight, but this weight loss will be a mix of fat and muscle tissue. As a result, your resting metabolic rate will decrease, which will make it more difficult to lose weight and keep it off over time. However, if you restrict your calories while also performing strength training, the weight you lose will be almost entirely fat tissue. This will allow you to maintain your resting metabolic rate, which will help to boost your ability to lose weight. However, in order to reap the benefits of boosting your metabolism from strength training, you'll need to design a program that follows the guidelines regarding frequency, intensity, and mode, as outlined by the American College of Sports Medicine[15].

Strength Training Program Guidelines

Perhaps the number one measure of a beneficial cardiovascular exercise routine is the cumulative length of your workouts over the course of a week. This is the case because the number of calories burned and the amount of time you spend in the "afterburn," the period in which your metabolism is elevated after your workout, are largely dependent on how long you spend exercising. On the other hand, when designing an effective strength-training program, the duration of your workout is practically irrelevant, as the most important factors to consider are frequency, intensity, and mode.

Frequency

As previously mentioned, when you perform strength-training exercises, you are creating microscopic tears in your muscles, which then heal to create additional muscle tissue. This process is what leads to muscle growth, an increase in your metabolism, and weight loss. In order for this process to work most effectively, your muscles need at least forty-eight hours of time in between strength-training sessions to heal. Otherwise, the tears you created during your previous workout will only become larger because they won't have time to heal, which will only deter muscle growth. Therefore, you should aim to create a strength-training program that allows for at least one day of rest in between working out the same muscle groups. This doesn't mean that you can't perform strength training each day, but if you do, you should ensure that you aren't exercising the same muscle groups on back-to-back days. For instance, you could make day one's workout focus on lower body exercises and day two's focus on upper body exercises, as one example. This type of schedule will create built-in time for your muscles to heal.

On the other side of the spectrum, you'll need to perform strength training at least twice a week in order to see results. If you choose to perform strength training twice a week, these two days should consist of full-body workouts, which means they should include exercises that work your chest, shoulders, arms, back, legs, and core muscles. This usually equates to at least eight to ten exercises.

Goal	Repetitions	Rest between sets
Strength Gains	4-8	2-3 minutes
Muscle Growth	8-12	60-90 seconds
Muscle Endurance	12-15	30-60 seconds

Intensity

Unlike cardiovascular exercise, the time that you spend performing strength training isn't that important; rather, you should put an emphasis on the number of sets and reps you perform. Studies have shown that significant strength gains can be made by performing just one set of strength training exercises and that these gains increase with the addition of an increased number of sets[16]. A general rule of thumb is to perform three sets of each exercise, but you will certainly derive benefit from performing one or two sets. How many sets you decide to incorporate into your routine should be based on how much time you have available to dedicate to strength training. However, the number of repetitions you decide to perform should be thought of differently.

The number of repetitions you decide to perform and the duration of rest in between sets should be based on the goals you want to achieve. The American College of Sports Medicine's guidelines, which you can use to align your goals with how many repetitions you decide to include, can be found here:

A good rule of thumb for determining how much resistance to use is to pick a resistance you feel very comfortable lifting for each exercise. Then in each subsequent workout, add a small amount of resistance. When you reach a level in which the last two repetitions begin to become a struggle to complete, this is when you know you've reached an adequate level of resistance. You should maintain this level of resistance until the last two repetitions become easier to complete, at which point you can resume adding small amounts of resistance.

Mode

Any mode, or in other words, any type of resistance you choose to employ in order to perform strength training will be effective as long as you are following the guidelines we just outlined regarding frequency and intensity. Your options for the type of resistance you can employ include but are not limited to dumbbells, cables, strength training machines, resistance bands, and bodyweight exercises. Your decision about what mode you choose should be based on factors such as access and convenience, but there is no wrong choice. In fact, you may choose to incorporate a variety of modes into your strength training routine.

Designing a Strength Training Routine Using ACSM's Frequency, Intensity, and Mode Guidelines

Okay, so now that you have guidance on how frequently, at what intensity, and what type of strength training exercises you should be performing in order to promote weight loss, let's look at some sample routines. Only you will be able to generate a routine that works best for you, but hopefully, these examples can help to give you a jumping-off point.

Example 1: Stacey

Stacey is a busy executive and a mother of two children under the age of five. Due to her hectic schedule, she has decided to perform two full-body strength-training sessions each week at home. On Tuesday, she performs strength training using tubing, and on Thursday, she streams a bodyweight strength training routine online. Her tubing exercise routine takes her fifteen minutes to complete, and the variety of strength training workouts she streams online lasts for twenty minutes each. This is what her weekly routine looks like:

Tuesday	Thursday
Tubing exercises that include two sets of:	Sample of the bodyweight exercises she performs during a streaming workout
Chest Fly	Push-ups
Back Row	Jump squats
Lateral Shoulder Raise	Reverse lunges
Front Shoulder Raise	Dips

Bicep Curls	Russian Twists
Triceps Kickback	Side Lunges
Squats	Bicycles
Lunges	Burpees
CORE exercises	Planks

Example 2: Mohamed

Mohamed is married, works as a researcher for a biotech company, and spends long hours at the office. In order to ensure that he fits in his strength training workouts, he lifts weights at home before going to work three days a week. Mohamed completes three sets of each exercise, which equates to about a half hour of strength training. Here is what his routine looks like:

Monday	**Wednesday**	**Friday**
Bench Press	Chest Fly	Incline Bench Press
Shoulder Press	Front Raise	Arnold Press

Lat Pulldown	Barbell Row	Reverse Fly
Bicep Curl	Hammer Curl	Straight Bar Curl
Squats	Lunges	Side Lunges
Overhead Triceps Press	Triceps Kickback	Bench Dips
Step-Ups with Dumbbell	Toe Raise	Side-Steps
Shrugs	Lateral Raise	Shrugs
CORE Circuit	Plank Circuit	CORE Circuit

Example 3: Michelle

Michelle is a single elementary school teacher who likes to de-stress by going to the gym after work, Monday through Thursday. Before hitting the treadmill, she likes to perform some strength-training exercises. She usually performs one to two sets of each exercise as a circuit in order to get through her routine in fifteen minutes or less. Here is what her routine looks like:

Monday	Tuesday	Wednesday	Thursday
Chest Press Machine	Leg Press Machine	Chest Press Machine	Leg Press Machine
Overhead Press Machine	Hip Abduction/Adduction Machine	Overhead Press Machine	Hip Abduction/Adduction Machine
Lateral Raise Machine	Biceps Curl Machine	Lateral Raise Machine	Biceps Curl Machine
Triceps Press Machine	Lat PullDown Cable	Triceps Press Machine	Lat PullDown Cable
Calf Raise Machine	Low Row Cable	Calf Raise Machine	Low Row Cable
Abdominal Crunch Machine	Back Extension Machine	Abdominal Crunch Machine	Back Extension Machine

Varying Intensity and Mode to Maximize Results

Now that you have a solid understanding of how to create an effective strength-training program that will work for you, I want to clarify that it is important to occasionally vary the intensity and mode of your workouts. The reason to add variety to the intensity and mode of your strength- training routine is that it will help you maximize your results.

Two things will happen if you continue to perform the same type of exercises at the same level of intensity for long periods of time. First, your body and your mind will get bored, which will lead to a plateau or, worse, complete disengagement. Second, even if you are the type of person who can perform the same routine at the same intensity for months on end, eventually, you'll start to develop overuse injuries. Therefore, it is good to vary your level of intensity and mode at least every twelve weeks.

By changing up your routine, you'll be able to stay mentally and physically engaged, and you'll avoid overuse injuries. In order to provide this type of variety, I'd recommend changing the types of exercises you are performing on a routine basis. The simplest way to do this is to change modalities, such as replacing free weight exercises with tubing exercises or replacing tubing exercises with bodyweight exercises. It could also simply equate to streaming a variety of strength training workouts instead of the same one over and over again. The other way to provide variety to your strength training routine is to periodically change the intensity.

The easiest way to change the intensity of your strength-training routine is to switch up the number of repetitions you perform. For instance, you might want to start by performing eight to twelve repetitions to maximize muscle growth in order to boost your resting metabolic rate. However, after twelve weeks, I'd recommend switching to twelve to fifteen repetitions in order to lower your intensity and reduce the burden on your joints while continuing to gain the benefits related to regular strength training.

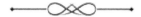

Katy: Strength training is one of those things that I know cognitively is a good idea, but I just always had a hard time getting it into my exercise rotation. Historically, this has been for a couple of reasons. First off, I really like the satisfaction I feel when I've worked out doing cardio. I **like** getting a lot of steps in on a run or a long walk. It feels good to rack up 10,000 or 15,000 steps in a day. I **like** seeing a long distance on a fitness tracker app on my phone. I can feel the satisfaction from completing an intense cardio workout almost immediately (whether through the buckets of sweat pouring off my body or through data in fitness apps). Doing strength training does have positive effects, but it just takes longer for me to notice and/or realize them. When I've had a good strength-training workout, I sweat a lot and have the spent feeling of exhausted muscles. But it's not usually until the next day (or the day after!) that I really feel the impact of muscle soreness and that delayed effect sometimes makes it harder to feel motivated to get strength training in on the regular. I have learned, over time, to appreciate the satisfaction of sore muscles the next day – but the delay in that satisfaction initially made it difficult for me to stay motivated to do the strength training in the first place.

Another reason it took awhile to get strength training regularly incorporated into my exercise routine was just a simple lack of know-how. I had **never** done any kind of strength training, weightlifting, resistance training, etc. Ever. I didn't have any equipment at home and had no idea where to start. At the gym, there were all kinds of weight machines available but I found them so intimidating, I wouldn't touch them. At the gym, I watched people confidently navigate the machines but didn't have the courage to ask for help learning how to use them. Luckily, because of Ryan's encouragement to intentionally incorporate strength training into my exercise routine, I finally mustered up the courage to sign up for one-on-one training with a personal trainer at my gym once per week. I started working with my personal trainer the following Saturday and I was **so** nervous. I explained to her that I felt good about what I was doing in terms of cardio but needed help establishing a regular routine of strength training. I felt clumsy and awkward and did not at all feel like I'd be able to do very much. She was unbelievably kind and patient with me and **started where I was**. After a brief assessment, it became quite clear that I had pretty poor core strength: I could hardly do a sit-up. She put me on an incline bench and asked me to roll up into a crunch and I couldn't make my body sit up. I was lying there partially upside down with no ability to get myself up, not unlike a turtle floundering on its shell. It was very sobering. By this time I could do a slow jog for a mile and yet I had no idea just how weak I really was.

She decided to start me off with very basic strength training options mostly using my own body weight as resistance. This was a perfect place for me to start. She taught me how to do several basic moves and never, ever, made me feel self-conscious when I wasn't sure what to do. I remember her genuine shock when I told her I had never done a squat before and wasn't sure how to do it. She just patiently demonstrated and helped me learn how to have good form while I did my first squat ever. She taught me how to do lunges, supermans, and leg lifts. In time, she introduced me to the weight machines at the gym and we started incorporating those into my half-hour sessions. I met with her once/week and then on at least two other days throughout the week, I would find a time to do the strength-training exercises she gave me to do. As I gained experience with the exercises, I became so much more confident on the machines and in the gym. I felt more and more like I belonged there and felt so much less fear about my ability to do things "right."This was a big step for me. I clearly remember the day that I excitedly sent my weekly email to Ryan and reported that I had actually independently used a weight machine. In my journey, I have learned not to minimize steps like this. In retrospect, it seems silly that I was so nervous about using the weight machines at the gym, but I assure you, in the moment, it didn't feel silly at all. It felt intimidating and overwhelming. Celebrating all the milestones, including this one, have been very important parts of my healthy weight-loss journey.

A few months after I'd been consistently doing strength training two to three days/week, my trainer at the gym asked me to get back on the incline bench. I couldn't understand why she wanted me to do it – the previous time she'd had me get on I had lain there totally stuck. Imagine my surprise when I curled up into a perfect crunch with almost no effort at all. I couldn't believe it! Doing all those exercises for all those months had managed to strengthen my core without my even being aware of it! That is the magic of strength training to me. It slowly builds muscle and ability and, in time, enables you to achieve feats you previously thought completely impossible. More recently, I have noticed how steady strength training has enabled me to be confident in outdoor adventures where I need to shimmy my body over rocks and/or in slot canyons on hikes in Southern Utah. It is an amazing thing to know my body is strong and capable and engaging in consistent strength training is what has enabled that.

What's Next?

Having finished reading this chapter, you should have a solid idea of how you can use regular strength training to boost your metabolism and maximize your weight loss results. You should also have a firm understanding of how to create a strength-training routine that will work for you. But remember, strength training is just one of many menu options that you will need to consider when designing your weight-loss plan. In the next and last section of this book, Create and Launch, you will design and implement your weight-loss plan by incorporating the wealth of knowledge that you have accumulated while reading the Explore section.

Chapter Nine Key Takeaways:

- Strength training is even more effective at promoting weight loss than cardiovascular exercise because of its positive effect on your resting metabolic rate.

- Performing regular strength training can increase your resting metabolic rate by as much as 7 percent.

- Performing regular strength training on its own can help you lose up to fifteen to twenty pounds over the course of a year.

- Losing weight solely through caloric restriction will cause you to lose muscle tissue, slow your metabolism, and stunt your weight loss efforts.

- At a minimum, strength training should be performed twice a week.

Phase Three: Create and Launch

Congratulations, you have made it to the planning phase! In this section, you will use the road map you developed in the Connect phase and the knowledge you acquired in the Explore phase to create an effective and sustainable weight-loss plan. By the time you finish the Create and Launch phase, you will be ready to hit the ground running with a weight loss plan that is going to work for you. In order to create this plan, you'll be taking a few final steps as you move through this section, including conducting a gap analysis, setting goals, and creating an accountability plan. Once you've completed these three steps, you'll launch your plan! So let's not waste another second and get to work on conducting your gap analysis.

Chapter 10

Conducting a Gap Analysis

Step 4: Conduct a Gap Analysis

As you'll recall, during steps one through three, you conducted a self-assessment, identified your personal values, and created your ideal wellness vision. Your next step is to compare how your current habits align with your desired future state by conducting a gap analysis.

If we were living a life in which our behaviors perfectly aligned with our personal values, then we would be living a life that was, well, perfect. The truth is that none of us are able to make 100 percent of our behaviors reflect our personal values 100 percent of the time, which is why the ideal wellness vision you created is a desired future state and not your current reality. However, the goal of this chapter is to help you identify where the largest discrepancies exist between your current behaviors and your ideal wellness vision. To pinpoint these discrepancies, you'll conduct something called a gap analysis.

A gap analysis is when you compare your actual performance to your desired future state. For your purposes, you'll be comparing your current health behaviors to your ideal wellness vision in order to determine where the "gaps" exist. Once these gaps have been identified, you'll be able to create goals to address these gaps, which, once achieved, will lead you to the achievement of your ideal wellness vision.

Conducting Your Gap Analysis

It is common knowledge that in order to achieve the desired vision, one must set goals, which, if achieved, will lead to the attainment of this vision. However, a critical but often overlooked step that must be taken before setting goals is to understand the discrepancy that exists between one's vision and their current reality. Understanding where the discrepancies lie will allow you to set meaningful and impactful goals. If you were to skip this step, you would be opening yourself up to the possibility that the goals you set, even if you achieved them, would not lead you to your ideal wellness vision.

In order to understand the discrepancy that exists between the vision you created for yourself and your current reality, you'll need to reflect back on **your** ideal wellness vision, your personal values, and your self-assessment. Once you have these items in hand and ready to review, please follow these three steps to conduct your gap analysis:

Step 1: Review and Edit (if necessary) Your Ideal Wellness Vision and Personal Values

The first step is to review the ideal wellness vision that you created for yourself and your list of personal values by asking yourself these questions:

Is this still the person I want to be one year from now?

Do these personal values represent what matters most to me in life?

If you answered no to either of these questions, please take a moment to edit your vision and your personal values until they reflect a future state that truly excites you and is representative of your personal values. Once your vision and list of personal values are ready to go, you'll need to identify which of your current behaviors are not in congruence with your vision by examining your self-assessment.

Step 2: Recognize What Is Already Going Well

To understand which areas have discrepancies between your ideal wellness vision and your current behaviors, you'll need to review your self-assessment. First, please take a moment to recognize all of the behaviors that you are already performing to support the future achievement of your ideal wellness vision. I bet there are more than you thought! You should be proud of these healthy behaviors that you are already performing, and if you think they are well ingrained into your life, you can leave them out of the planning process. But before moving on, please pause to give yourself a pat on the back for the healthy habits you are already practicing. Well done!

Step 3: Identify the Gaps

Now that you have identified what you are already doing well, it's time to take a look at the areas in which you think you have the most room to improve. To do this, please review your self-assessment and write down each behavior that, if changed, would bring you closer towards your ideal wellness vision on your plan template. Please take note that if you see a behavior that, if changed, would bring you closer to your ideal wellness vision, but you currently have no intention of changing, don't add it to your list. Remember, you should only make behavioral changes when you are ready to do so; otherwise, they will be dead on arrival.

Once your list is complete, think back to the chapters you just read in the Explore phase in order to prioritize which behaviors, if changed, would help you make the biggest leaps towards your ideal wellness vision. Prioritize your list by assigning a ranking to each potential behavior change in the table provided as part of your planning template. Assign a ranking by using a one to five scale, with five representing the most impactful and one representing the least impactful behavior change.

Interpreting Your Gap Analysis

You certainly don't have to be Einstein to interpret your gap analysis results. The behavior changes with the highest numerical ranking are the ones that you believe, if changed, would allow you to close the gap that exists between your current reality and your ideal wellness vision.

Katy: After spending the time and energy to identify a vision for yourself, assessing your current state of behaviors that are either contributing or not contributing to your health, and learning all the different facets that contribute to a healthy lifestyle, you've made it to the fun part! You get to start assembling an action plan that, step-by-step will lead you to the lifestyle you really want for yourself. As Ryan points out, the first part of building an actionable plan is figuring out where there is a disconnect between what you **say/believe** you want for yourself and what your lifestyle choices are allowing. This has not always been an easy process for me. I have found that while I am aware of some of my behaviors that are clearly creating a gap between where I am and where I ultimately want to be, other behaviors that create gaps have been harder for me to identify and address because of blind spots that I'm not even aware of. Completing the self-assessment with full honesty with yourself will, I believe, make this process easier.

Because it took me awhile to really settle on a solid vision for myself, it took me awhile to identify the gaps or barriers that were preventing me from the life I wanted. How do I know what behaviors are keeping me from the life I want if I don't actually know what life I want?? As you begin your gap analysis, I would echo Ryan and encourage you to take the time to review your wellness vision – you've probably had some new insights or maybe gotten some ideas as you've been reading the past few chapters. Perhaps there are ways you want to adjust your wellness vision. Are there ways in which you can now envision your life that you weren't able to previously? Are there things you want for your life that you hadn't been able to consider before? Be bold and be brave – this is **your** life and you can choose what you want it to look like! Perhaps your vision is still clear to you and it hasn't changed. Good for you! Regardless of how you get to it, a clearly-defined vision will help make the next steps manageable and actionable.

Identifying the areas I struggled with was a complex process for me. There were some areas that were glaringly obvious and others that were a bit more obscure. I **knew** that I had difficulty avoiding sugar and sweets, and I knew that difficulty was likely contributing to my inability to achieve some of the lifestyle (and specifically, the ideal weight) I envisioned (it was). I also knew that I wasn't great at managing stress without eating unhealthy or copious amounts of food. These were areas that I had struggled with for a long time and have taken (and continue to take) a lot of work and effort to address and manage. You probably have areas of your life like that too – but they may very well differ than my areas of struggle.

Of course, there were other areas of my self-assessment that led me to gaps I had not previously acknowledged. When I got to the section asking about how often I did strength training and stretching exercises, it shined a light on a whole area of fitness I had never even considered before. This was a gap that I simply had overlooked and the self-assessment helped me to understand that, while I was consistently exercising, to achieve my ideal wellness vision, it was going to be important that I expand the type of exercise I was including in my daily routine. This blind spot came about as a result of a lack of knowledge. You may find some of those blind spots in your own life and, once you learn more, you can address them.

The self-assessment also led to the discovery of other blind spots I was completely unaware of. Although I knew that I struggled with eating well when I got stressed, I had never stopped to consider what other habits I had in my life that were contributing to this particular weakness. On the self-assessment, I discovered two important areas that I had never connected to my difficulty with stress eating. I reported that: 1) I rarely used daily strategies (i.e., breathing, stretching, relaxation, imagery, meditation) to manage stress; and 2) I rarely released anxiety, worry, and fear in a healthy way. Although it seems obvious to me now, at the time, I just failed to connect that perhaps the reason I was vulnerable to eating when I was stressed was because I had not developed other strategies to manage my stress in a healthy way. This discovery led to intentionally incorporating time for personal meditation every day. It helped contribute to my decision to seek help from a mental health therapist who helped me learn strategies to better manage anxiety. A thoughtful consideration of how the areas you are struggling with may be contributing to a gap between where you are and where you want to be is rather empowering.

What's Next?

So, you are ready to start setting goals in order to change these behaviors, right? Not so fast; first, you must identify which stage of change you are currently in for each identified behavior. Otherwise, it would be like trying to turn a seedling into a plant without knowing what type of vegetation you were trying to help grow. In the next chapter, you will identify the stage of change you are in for each behavior and write corresponding goals.

Chapter Ten Key Takeaways:

- Conducting a gap analysis allows you to identify the discrepancies that exist between your desired future state and your current behaviors.

- The results of your gap analysis will allow you to prioritize potential behavior changes.

Chapter Ten To-Do List:

Before reading Chapter 11, please make sure that you have completed each of these actions and added them to your planning template:

✓ Identify the gaps that exist between your current behaviors and your ideal wellness vision.

✓ Create a list of the behaviors that, if changed, would help you close this gap by examining the results of your self-assessment.

✓ Prioritize your behavior change list by assigning each one a ranking on a one to five scale.

Chapter 11

Goal Setting

Hundreds of books have been written about the topic of goal setting and for a good reason. Nearly every success story starts with a person setting a goal. Certainly, the achievement of your ideal wellness vision would qualify as a success story, and like many others' stories, the creation of goals will lay the foundation for your future success.

The most effective way to write a goal is by using the S.M.A.R.T. (specific, measurable, achievable, relevant, and time-bound) goal-setting method. In addition to making your goals S.M.A.R.T. goals, we are going to supercharge them by including two other key elements: your stage of change and positivity-based goal setting.

After you have read this chapter, you will understand the Transtheoretical Model of Change and will be able to explain the difference between positive and negative-based goals. You will have also put this knowledge to use by setting a three-month outcome and behavioral goals for yourself. Although I'm sure you're eager to start setting your goals, it is important to decide what *type* of change you are ready to make before launching into goal setting; in order to decide what type of change you are ready to make, you'll need to have an understanding of the Transtheoretical Model of Behavior Change.

Transtheoretical Model of Behavior Change

This model was developed by Prochaska and DiClemente in the late 1970s and focused on the decision-making of the individual. Prochaska and DiClemente's research, which focused on individuals who were trying to quit smoking, found that people do not change behaviors quickly and decisively, but rather change occurs continuously through a cyclical process. Although their initial research was focused on smoking cessation, the stages of change they identified can be applied to any type of behavior change, including the adoption of behaviors that lead to successful and sustainable weight loss. This cycle of behavior change can be mapped to five different stages of change; precontemplation, contemplation, preparation, action, and maintenance.

- *Precontemplation* – In the precontemplation stage, people do not intend to take action within the next six months. Often people are unaware or in denial that there is a reason to change or they would like to, but they don't believe change is possible. Terms in this stage that are often used are: "I won't or I can't." People in this stage are not yet ready to set behavior change goals.

- *Contemplation* – In this stage, people are ready to make a change within the next six months. They recognize that their behavior may be problematic and can see the advantages of making a change. The term most used in this stage is "I may." People in this stage should set goals related to further research and/or "thinking" goals (i.e., searching for gyms close to home, reading articles about healthy breakfasts, talking with a spouse about what type of exercise schedule may work best for both of their schedules, etc.).

213

- *Preparation* – In the preparation stage, people are ready to take action within the next thirty days. People in this stage believe that changing their behavior can lead to a healthier life. The term most used by people in this stage is "I will." For people in this stage of change, they should set goals related to specific preparation that needs to take place prior to action (i.e., purchasing sneakers, signing up for a gym membership, downloading an app to track their calories, purchasing a scale, etc.).

- *Action* – In this stage, people have changed their behavior within the last six months and plan to keep moving forward with that behavior change. People in this stage believe in the importance of adopting healthier behaviors and display actions that support this belief. The term used most often by people in this stage is "I am." People in this stage should set goals that exhibit actionable behavior (i.e. – run for thirty minutes three times a week, eat five servings of vegetables seven days a week, get into bed no later than 10:00 p.m. every night, etc.).

- *Maintenance* – In the maintenance stage, people have sustained their behavior change for more than six months and intend to maintain the behavior change going

- forward. People in this stage most often use the term "I still am" to describe their actions. People in this stage of change should set goals that support the continuation of the healthy behavior they have adopted and that protect against relapsing to earlier stages (i.e., continue to run for thirty minutes three days a week, continue to eat five servings of vegetables seven days a week).

When considering setting goals for yourself, you should always match the stage of change you are in with the type of goal you are setting in order to maximize your results. If you fail to coordinate the type of goal you set with the stage of change you are in, the likelihood that you won't achieve your goal increases greatly. In order to have the greatest level of success, you should set goals for yourself that match the stage you are in within the Transtheoretical Model, as outlined in the table below:

Stage of Change	Goal Type	Goal Example
Pre-contemplation	Do not set a goal at this time	n/a
Contemplation	Thinking goal	Decide what days of the week I will exercise by January 9th.
Preparation	Planning goal	Map out a two-mile walking route near my office that I can utilize on my lunch break by January 16th.
Action	Action goal	Take a two-mile walk during my lunch break on January 26th.
Maintenance	Continuation goal	Continue to take a two-mile walk on my lunch break on Monday, Wednesday, and Friday each week.

Now that you have a grasp on the Transtheoretical Model of Behavioral Change and how it relates to goal setting, please add the stage of change you are in for each of the behaviors you identified during your gap analysis to your planning template. After you have completed this step, it is time to learn about positivity-based goal setting.

Positivity-Based Goal Setting

How you think about a goal can influence whether you achieve it or not. If you are excited about executing your goal, then the likelihood that you will achieve it goes up exponentially. On the flip side, if the goal you have created makes you wince, then chances are you aren't going to have much success. One way to ensure that your goals are written in a way that makes you feel good about them is to keep them positive and avoid setting negativity-based or deprivation goals.

Goals can either be written using a positive or negative tense, or in other words, they can be set as approach or avoidance goals. For example, in order to lose weight, one of your intentions may be to eat a healthier diet. A positive tense/approach goal may read something like "eat at least five servings of fruits and vegetables per day," while a negative tense/avoidance goal would read something like "eat dessert no more than two nights a week." In simple terms, these goals are helping you achieve the same thing, a healthier diet, but the way in which they are written can influence how likely you are to achieve them.

In the example above, the avoidance goal is focused on *depriving* yourself of something you want, in this case, dessert. While on the other hand, the approach goal is focused on the *desired action*, to eat more fruits and vegetables. Avoidance goals are emotionally unappealing, which makes it difficult to focus on them and to be excited about achieving them. Setting goals in the positive tense will help you focus on success and will facilitate yourself envisioning your desired future state. Let's look at some other examples of positive vs. negative-based goals:

Desire	Positive (approach) goal	Negative (avoidance) goal
Reduce sugar intake	Drink at least eight glasses of water each day.	Limit myself to two cans of soda a week.
Improve sleep	Unwind by taking a bath before bed on Monday and Wednesday evenings each week.	Eliminate all screen use by 7 p.m. each night.
Exercise more often	Ride my bike to work at least three days a week.	Only drive my car to work twice a week.

With an understanding of the Transtheoretical Model of Behavior Change and positivity-based goal-setting under your belt, you are now ready to start setting goals. To do so, you'll use the S.M.A.R.T. goal setting method.

S.M.A.R.T. Goal Setting

S.M.A.R.T. is an acronym that stands for specific, measurable, achievable, relevant, and time-bound. S.M.A.R.T. is an effective tool that provides the clarity, focus, and motivation you need to achieve your goals. Using this method can also improve your ability to reach your goals by encouraging you to define your objectives and set a completion date. S.M.A.R.T. goals have become widely used by individuals and corporations all over the world; however, not everyone is familiar with this form of goal setting, or some of you might need a refresher, which is why we will review the methodology here:

- Specific – If your goal is unclear or not specific enough, you won't be able to focus your efforts or feel motivated to achieve your goal. To ensure specificity when writing a goal, answer the following "w" questions:

  o **What** do I want to accomplish?

  o **Who** is involved?

  o **Where** is it located?

  o **Which** back-up plans do I need to put in place?

- Measurable – If your goal is not measurable, it is impossible to track your progress or measure your rate of success. Assessing progress helps you to stay focused and generates excitement when you are getting closer to achieving your goal. For a goal to be measurable, it should be able to answer questions like:

  o How many?

  o How often?

- o For how long?

- o For what distance?

- **A**chievable – Your goals must also be realistic and attainable in order for you to have success. In other words, your goal needs to be in your "sweet spot." This means it should be hard enough to achieve that it would make you excited if you accomplished it but realistic enough that the habit changes you make to achieve the goal are sustainable. If your goal is written to be achievable, it should be able to answer the following questions:

  - o How realistic is the goal, based on your other obligations/constraints?

  - o Is this goal sustainable?

  - o Would accomplishing this goal excite me?

- **R**elevant – If your goal is relevant, it should be in alignment with your vision. All of the goals you set, if achieved, should help to bring you one step closer to your ideal wellness vision. In order to ensure relevance when setting a goal, ask yourself the following questions:

  - o If I achieve this goal, will it bring me closer to my ideal wellness vision?

  - o What about this goal is meaningful to me?

- **Time-bound** – Every goal needs a target date; without a deadline, there is no sense of urgency for you to achieve the goal. Additionally, making your goals time-bound helps to prevent everyday tasks from taking priority over your longer-term goals. Through my research, I have found three target date ranges to be the most effective:

  o Long-term vision (1 year)

  o Medium range goals (3 months)

  o Short term goals (2 weeks)

As you can see, S.M.A.R.T. goal setting requires you to drill down on your goals in order to make your approach rock-solid. To make sure you have a handle on S.M.A.R.T. goal setting, let's review a concrete example.

Example: Marcus wants to eat a healthier breakfast

Marcus has identified through his gap analysis that he would benefit from eating a high protein breakfast. He currently eats breakfast each day, but it usually consists of cereal or a breakfast bar; both options offer less than 10 grams of protein. Let's examine his first attempt to set a goal and how he refined this goal to make it fit into the S.M.A.R.T. methodology and meet the positivity-based goal-setting criteria.

Initial goal attempt: Reduce cereal intake by eating a high protein breakfast three days a week.

At first glance, this looks like a decent goal, as it supports his efforts to increase his protein intake at breakfast. But what could be changed to improve this goal and increase Marcus's likelihood of success? First, every goal statement should be based on positivity, which means Marcus should remove the deprivation piece of this goal: *reduce cereal intake.*

> *Reduce cereal intake by eating a high protein breakfast three days a week.*

Next, Marcus should make this goal more specific and measurable by including how much protein he will eat at breakfast, what types of foods he will eat too in order to reach these metrics, and on what days of the week he will eat a high protein breakfast. Without knowing more about Marcus and his ideal wellness vision, it is hard to decipher if this goal is achievable and relevant, so let's assume it is. Finally, Marcus needs to put a deadline on achieving this goal so that he knows when to review his progress. By applying these changes, here is what Marcus's revised goal looks like:

> *Revised goal: Eat at least 15 grams of protein for breakfast by choosing to eat a Greek yogurt, two scrambled eggs made with skim milk, or a protein smoothie on Monday, Wednesday, and Friday mornings, over each of the next two weeks.*

Can you see how Marcus would be much more likely to achieve the revised goal? I sure can! One thing you might have noticed as part of Marcus's revised goal was he didn't specify what type of food he would be eating on a particular day. This was purposeful, as no one wants to feel like they are locked into eating eggs when they are in the mood for a refreshing smoothie. This type of hyper specificity is often much too aggressive and can lead to unhappiness and push-back. I am always an advocate for giving yourself menu options, especially if each option still leads you to your ultimate goal, which in this case, it does. Every option Marcus gave himself supports the consumption of at least 15 grams of protein for breakfast.

Making your goals S.M.A.R.T., while also building in goal flexibility are hallmarks of a well- written behavioral goal. As you may recall, every weight-loss plan should include a mix of outcome and behavioral goals. Way back in Chapter Three, you created a one-year weight loss outcome goal as part of your ideal wellness vision. In the next section of this chapter, you will identify the behavioral goals, which, if instituted, will lead you to the achievement of your outcome goal.

Behavioral Goal Setting

Let's examine goal setting by using the analogy of planning a road trip. When planning a road trip, your outcome goal would be your "destination," and your behavioral goals would be the "directions" you'll use to navigate there. The fun/easy part of planning a road trip is deciding where you are going to end up. The more challenging part of the planning process is figuring out how you will get there, where you will stay along the way, where you will eat, and your budget. However, without making these plans in advance, your trip is likely to go off course, or you may never even make it to your destination. This is why it is so critical to set behavioral goals which, if achieved, will lead you to your desired outcome goal.

When setting behavioral goals, you should make sure they are: in support of your outcome goals, match the stage of change you are currently in for each particular behavior, written using the S.M.A.R.T. format, and written in a positive tense. You'll need to keep these criteria in mind when creating your three-month goals.

Setting Your Three-Month Outcome and Behavioral Goals

Three-Month Outcome Goal

In order to set a three-month outcome goal, start by revisiting your one-year ideal wellness vision to determine what outcome you plan to achieve twelve months from now. Is your one-year outcome goal written in terms of pounds lost, inches lost, or both? Depending on your answer, please read one or both of the following sections:

Three-Month Outcome Goal: Pounds Lost

When setting an outcome goal related to weight loss, the most common metric used is pounds lost. This is the case because it is the easiest to track, all you need is a scale, and it is the simplest to predict due to the caloric deficit formula that you now know and love. When setting a three-month weight-loss goal, the simplest thing to do is to take the total amount of weight you plan to lose in a year and divide it by four. However, I would recommend front-loading your weight loss goals during the first three to six months, as this is the time frame in which you will most likely be at your peak level of motivation. I'd also recommend that you consider the following pacing guidelines.

- When setting a weight-loss goal using the metric of pounds per week, a good rule of thumb for most people is to set a goal of losing one pound per week.

- If your BMI is greater than 35, you might consider setting a more aggressive goal of 1.5–2 lbs a week (no more than 2 lbs).

- If your BMI is under 25, you may consider a less aggressive goal of .5 pounds per week.

Of course, these are just guidelines, and you should use your past experiences around weight loss and the knowledge you have about your own body to set an outcome goal that is the most appropriate for you. Once you have considered these guidelines and your own past experiences, please add a three-month weight-loss goal to your planning template.

Measurement Tip: I'd recommend that anyone who is using a scale to track their progress only weigh themselves once a week. This weigh-in should ideally take place in the morning, after using the bathroom but prior to eating or drinking, and should be done on the same day every week. Following these practices is the best way to gain an accurate measure of your progress. Weighing yourself more than once a week can lead to misleading perceptions of your progress (or lack thereof) as fluctuations in water weight, up and down, can lead you to dramatic inaccuracies.

Three-Month Outcome Goal: Inches Lost

Setting a weight loss goal by using the metric of pounds lost doesn't work well for everyone. Some people dread getting on a scale or find it really challenging not to weigh themselves more than once a week. In these cases, setting a goal around losing inches off of your waist may be a better fit for you. If this is the outcome measure you choose to track, there are a few things to consider when setting a goal for yourself. First, you'll want to understand what a realistic pace is for losing inches off your waist. Research tells us that, on average, for every 8.5 pounds lost, people dropped an inch off their waist. This means that every 10 pounds lost were accompanied by 1.18 inches of waistline reduction[1]. Therefore, as an example, if you believe it is reasonable to lose 1 pound a week over the course of twelve weeks, your outcome goal might be to reduce your waist circumference by 1.4 inches. However, you should use this formula to set a three-month goal around inches lost off your waist that is realistic yet exciting to you.

Pounds Lost	Inches Lost off of Waist
5	.59
10	1.18
15	1.77
20	2.36
25	2.95

When setting a three-month waist circumference goal, the simplest thing to do is to take the total number of inches you plan to lose in a year and divide it by four. However, just like when setting a goal related to pounds lost, I would recommend front-loading the inches you plan to lose during the first three to six months of your plan, as this is the time frame when you are likely to be strongly motivated.

Measurement Tip: Another thing you must consider when setting a goal related to inches lost is how you will ensure an accurate measurement of your waist circumference. To do so, I would recommend following these steps:

- Use a soft tape measure, the kind that is designed for a tailor or seamstress.

- Take your shirt off and stand in front of a mirror.

- Wrap the tape measure loosely around your waist, using your belly button as a marker.

- Take a deep breath in and let it out.

- After exhaling, tighten the tape measure around your belly button and put your finger on where the tape measure overlaps.

- The measurement where your finger is placed indicates your waist circumference.

Three Month Behavioral Goal Setting

Now that you have created three-month outcome goals, your "destination" has been identified, and it is time to draw up your set of "directions" on how to get there. These directions will consist of a set of three to five behavioral goals. To create your three-month behavioral goals, please follow these three steps:

Step 1: Review the table that you created within your planning template that illustrates the behaviors you'd like to change, the impact you believe they will have on helping you achieve your ideal wellness vision and the stage of change you are in for each behavior.

Step 2: Pick no less than three but no more than five of these behaviors to turn into three months S.M.A.R.T. goals that you believe will help you achieve the three-month outcome goal that you just set for yourself.

In order to decide which goals to pick, refer to the table you created to help you choose behaviors that would have the greatest impact and that you are most ready to change.

Step 3: Add these three to five behavioral goals to your planning template.

To get a sense of what someone else's three-month plan looks like, let's examine how Katy's planning template at this stage:

Behavioral Goals:

1. Perform at least 90 minutes of cardiovascular exercise 3 days/week.

Accountability Plan:

Potential barriers:

Back-up plans:

Stage of change: Action

2. Track all of the food I eat 7 days a week using a digital app

Accountability Plan:

Potential barriers:

Back-up plans:

Stage of change: Preparation

3. Plan 3 meals that include lean protein, whole grains, and vegetables, each week before going to the grocery store

Accountability Plan:

Potential barriers:

Back-up plans:

Stage of change: Preparation

4. 5 nights a week, eat a dinner consisting of a plate made up of ½ fruits/vegetables, ¼ protein, ¼ carbohydrate

Accountability Plan:

Potential barriers:

Back-up plans:

Stage of change: Preparation

5.Perform 10-15 minutes of strength training at least twice a week

Accountability Plan:

Potential barriers:

Back-up plans:

Stage of change: Contemplation

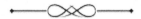

Katy: If you're like me, perhaps you've had a complicated relationship with goals over the course of your life. In the past, it wasn't uncommon for me to think big only to disappoint myself by my inability to meet my own grandiose expectations. Usually, the rollercoaster would look something like this:

- ✓ Be inspired to accomplish some great feat
- ✓ Feel super gungho and make an overwhelming plan
- ✓ Come out of the gate strong and feel really good about myself
- ✓ A couple of days in, begin to feel weighed down and overwhelmed by the task at hand
- ✓ Feel like I'm working hard but making little progress
- ✓ Make a seemingly valid excuse to depart from the overall plan
- ✓ Realize I'm not following the plan very well anymore
- ✓ Berate myself for not being able to achieve my goals
- ✓ Repeat. Repeat. Repeat.

As I look back, I now realize that <u>setting</u> goals was not the problem – I was a chronic setter of goals. I existed squarely in the Contemplation and Planning stages of Goal Setting. Thinking about and coming up with goals was motivating and exciting to me. Setting goals put me in the realm of endless possibilities for change. And I **loved** the possibility of change. Actually changing, however, required executing those goals. And things seemed to fall apart when it came to the execution stage. If setting goals and thinking of goals wasn't the problem, why was I struggling so much to make any active change toward accomplishing my health goals?

Ryan talked about the different stages of goal setting. When he initially taught me about these different stages, I knew I was already quite skilled at the contemplation stage. I regularly contemplated all the aspects of my health I wanted to change and how I wanted to improve. I did this so much that it sometimes got overwhelming! It took me some time to work out how to move out of the contemplation stage and translate that contemplation into goals that were actually actionable. This process led to the need to learn how to identify and articulate goals I could actually achieve. I established a principle I now regularly live by: I do not set a goal unless I **know** I can achieve it. That might sound overly simplistic but this is a rule of thumb that has worked well for me. For me, **knowing** I can achieve a goal means a few things. First, it means that my goal has to have a clear end. I don't set goals like "I will get healthy" or "I will lose a lot of weight" because neither of those declarations have a clear endpoint. How do I know exactly when I have "gotten healthy," or how much exactly is "a lot" of weight? By adhering to the principles around writing S.M.A.R.T. goals, I am much more likely to generate a goal that is measurable and has a clear end that tells me when I have achieved it. Such goals that I have specifically set included:

✓ I will walk at least three miles on five days/wk for six weeks in a row.

231

✓ I will stay within my calorie budget every day for seven days straight.

✓ I will plank for one whole minute.

✓ I will go on forty hikes this year."

Second, <u>knowing</u> I can achieve a goal means that I set goals that I even want to achieve in the first place. This one has taken some practice for me. It has required me to really consider what things I want to do in my life and to ignore influences that may dictate what others say I "should" do. With the influence of social media, it's very easy to see what everyone else is doing and get caught up in feeling we should be setting certain kinds of goals. It can be hard to resist the social pressure of these goals, but it has been very important for me to consider the goals I want to achieve independent of what everyone else is doing. A few years ago, I felt the vast majority of people I admired were off running marathons (it wasn't true; the seemingly "vast majority" was actually like six people . . .). I admired their achievements and was impressed they accomplished the amazing physical feat of running over twenty-six miles. In a row! Is it a good thing to run a marathon? Sure! Did I really want to run one myself? No, not really. But I felt kind of dumb for setting what felt like a piddly goal by comparison to running a marathon: I wanted to run a 5K. It took some time for me to realize that it really doesn't matter what anyone else's goals are – I needed to seriously think about what I wanted for me in **my** life. When I set that goal to run a 5K, I couldn't run for more than about a quarter of a mile at a time. While running a marathon felt unachievable to me, running a 5K felt like a manageable (and still challenging!) goal to achieve. I set the goal, started working toward it, and six months later I managed to do it! My next goal was to run a 10K. You may be thinking, "And then she set a goal to do a half-marathon! And then a marathon!" Nope. I ran my 10K and then decided I was ready for a new goal that didn't involve running. It turns out that, right now, that's about as far as I'm interested in taking my running journey. And that's okay. This isn't to say that someday I won't take on a marathon, but at this point, I don't have any plans to do so. I have other goals I'm gunning for and that feels fine to me. To me, goals are personal and should be tailored to the things that **you** want to achieve. I've set and achieved other physical goals: to ride my bike for 150 miles over two days; to summit a mountain; to swim a mile.

I have learned to really love setting goals. They contribute to a process of change that, in my life, has led me to places I never would have dreamed possible. And that is the real magic of goals. I mentioned that my rule of thumb is to only set goals that are achievable. What's so neat about goals is that, over time, as you achieve your goals, once unachievable goals become completely possible. The very first S.M.A.R.T. goal that I set and achieved was a very simple one. I simply set a goal to go for a walk five days/week for six weeks. I didn't put any constraints on the distance or intensity of those walks. My only stipulation was that it had to be beyond my regular daily activities (e.g., I couldn't count walking from my car into my work building as my 'walk'). At that time, I weighed 315 pounds and led a pretty sedentary life. Going for a walk every day fit every criteria Ryan talks about for setting goals: it was specific (go for a walk beyond my daily routine), measurable (did I walk? Yes or no?), achievable (I wasn't ready to run yet, but I could definitely walk!), relevant (I wanted to increase activity in my life, and it was time-bound (I wanted to do it for six weeks).

When I achieved that initial goal, I changed one aspect of it: I specified an actual distance and decided to walk for at least two miles. Once I achieved that two-mile walk every day goal, I changed another aspect: I decided to walk for three miles at a time. Eventually, I started adding and altering the goal in other ways: I made it longer, I added jogging, I did a morning **and** an afternoon walk. Achieving each goal in turn got me to a place where I could achieve other goals. I continue to be so proud of myself for setting that very first seemingly small goal. Several years later, after I had achieved enough goals that I was physically in totally different shape, my weight was down by 140 pounds, I was doing almost any physical activity I set out to do, I set a goal to hike a mountain in Utah, a state I had just moved to. This was a big goal for me. I would be hiking approximately 15 miles in one day and climbing over 5000 feet in elevation. I knew it would be hard and I was nervous about my ability to do it. But, I had achieved so many previous goals I was confident I **could** achieve it. I put in the work and I trained for the hike by doing a lot of smaller hikes, running, and conditioning myself the best I could. As I summited the peak, high above the valley below, I could not stop the tears from flowing as I considered not only the physical mountain of earth I had just conquered but the mental/emotional/physical mountain journey to get my health to where it was.

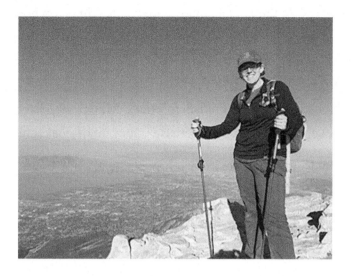

When I started those daily walks at 315 pounds there was **no way** I could have envisioned that I would be able to hike that mountain or weigh 170 pounds. Had I told my original self that that's where I would be in a few short years, I would have openly scoffed at the idea. But, the fact is, I **did** get there! How? By small and simple goals. And as you set S.M.A.R.T. achievable goals, you'll be surprised where they will lead you too. I can't wait to see where my road continues to lead me. I'm still setting goals. I've still got new mountains, literal and figurative, to climb.

What's Next?

As I'm sure you can tell by the progression of your planning template, your weight-loss plan is nearly ready to be set in motion. However, you still have a few really important additions to make to your plan, including accountability systems, the identification of barriers, and back-up plans. In the next chapter, your focus will be on how to build systems of accountability into your weight-loss plan.

Chapter Eleven Key Takeaways:

- Considering the Transtheoretical Model of Change when developing goals will increase your rate of goal achievement.

- Goals that are positive/approach based are more effective than goals that are negative/avoidance based.

- Goals written in the S.M.A.R.T. format are more likely to be achieved.

Chapter Eleven To-Do List:

Before reading Chapter Twelve, please make sure that you have completed each of these actions and added them to your planning template:

- ✓ Establish a three-month outcome goal.

- ✓ Create three to five, three-month behavioral goals.

Chapter 12

Accountability

I started working at my first job when I was fifteen years old. It was a summer job working for the municipal department of public works maintaining a local park. Me and another boy my age would spend our days weed whacking, picking up trash, and doing whatever minor maintenance jobs needed to be done. We were both excited to have jobs and worked diligently for the first several weeks of the summer. However, this diligence started to wane as the weeks went on primarily because there wasn't a system of accountability built into our jobs. Our boss would tell us what needed to be done each Monday, and then we wouldn't see him again until the following week. Additionally, no one was checking to see if the tasks assigned to us were actually completed.

This complete lack of accountability did not help to promote a successful and efficient workweek, especially for two fifteen-year-old kids. Now, did we continue to work? Of course, but we stretched our assignments out over the duration of the week and built-in plenty of time to relax and socialize with our other friends who were working at a nearby summer camp. Looking back on this experience, I have a couple of reflections. First, what a perfect first job; talk about easing into the workforce! Second, as a teenager asked to do manual labor, I would have benefited from a more stringent system of accountability. However, during other parts of my life, while working in different roles, a weekly check-in would have been more than enough accountability. This variance in the amount/type of accountability we need as people is dependent upon the circumstances surrounding the task and our level of intrinsic motivation.

Yes, I could have used frequent accountability to make sure I was working efficiently at my first summer job, but in other circumstances, I needed far less accountability. For example, I was very motivated to write this book because I knew it had the potential to help so many people, and I would have written it no matter what. However, partnering with Katy as a co-author helped to create a sense of urgency that wouldn't have otherwise existed. After we decided to author this book together, Katy and I checked in with each other twice a month by phone. During these phone calls, we would verbally commit to achieving certain writing goals, and then we would follow-up on the progress we made during our next call. Without this accountability plan, this book might still be just an idea or at best, still be unfinished.

When considering your weight-loss plan, you will probably require different levels/forms of accountability for each of your behavioral goals. For instance, you may be very intrinsically motivated to exercise and therefore, will only need to create a self-accountability plan for goals related to exercise. While on the other hand, you may be less intrinsically motivated to make changes to your diet and, as a result, will decide to set up a more rigorous accountability plan when setting goals related to improving your eating habits. In this chapter, we'll review different forms and levels of accountability so that you can decide what type(s) and intensity of accountability to build into your plan.

Accountability can come in various forms, and each individual will require different levels of accountability to support the achievement of their various goals. Although there are many variables to consider, there is no doubt that utilizing accountability positively impacts goal achievement. In fact, The American Society of Training and Development (A.S.T.D.) conducted a study on accountability and found that people have a 65 percent chance of completing a goal if they commit to someone other than themselves. Furthermore, if they made an accountability appointment with someone, there was an increase in their rate of goal achievement by up to 95 percent.

Clearly, accountability can be a powerful tool to employ when setting goals. However, not every person will need to utilize outside accountability for every goal they set. Often a person is able to set numerous goals, commit to doing them only to themselves, and achieve the goals. But there are definitely times when a person will know right from the jump that they need to utilize outside accountability in order to help them achieve their goal, or they may try to achieve the goal without using accountability and decide after a period of trial and error that the use of accountability could really help them.

As part of your plan, I'll ask you to assign a form (or more) of intrinsic or extrinsic accountability to each one of your three-month goals. With that said, I'll, of course, ask you to decide what type of accountability strategy will work best for each of your goals. The forms of accountability that are most commonly used are: boosted self-accountability, family/friends, and organized support. We'll review each of these strategies so that you can decide which one(s) you'd like to incorporate into your plan.

Boosted Self-Accountability

The simplest form of accountability is holding yourself accountable for your actions. For some individuals, for certain types of goals, mentally stating to themselves that they are going to follow through on action is enough to ensure that the goal will be accomplished. However, oftentimes a more intense level of accountability is necessary in order to ensure success.

Boosted levels of self-accountability can come in the form of verbal commitments, written commitments, the use of visual reminders, and/or technology-based reminders. Stating your goals out loud or writing them down helps to enhance your brain's encoding process, which is what helps you analyze and remember your goals. Neuroscience has shown that individuals are more likely to remember the material they've generated themselves as compared to material that they've read or heard. Therefore, when you speak your goals out loud or, even better, write them down, you're forcing your brain to regenerate the goal you created in your mind and, as a result, imprint it more firmly into your memory. As you can tell, verbally stating and writing down your goals can have a positive impact on how likely you are to remember and act on your goals. To create a second layer of support, you can add external reminders to your plan.

With the busy lives that we all lead, sometimes verbally stating and writing down your goals just isn't enough to keep your intentions in the forefront of your mind. However, using visual reminders, calendar alerts, or apps can all be used to keep you on track. When my wife and I set a goal to purchase a house, I created a visual reminder of our goal and put it on our refrigerator. My little poster had a thermometer, the kind you see organizations use for fundraising drives, with the amount of money we needed to save in order to purchase our next house at the top, and we could color in areas every time we saved $1,000. My poster also had pictures of a farmer's porch, a fireplace, and a jacuzzi tub, as reminders of what we envisioned as part of our next house. These pictures served as reminders of why it was worth saving our money to make the thermometer rise instead of spending it on other things. Each time my wife and I looked at the poster, it served as a reminder of our goal.

I've also leveraged technology such as calendar reminders and apps to remind me of my goals and/or to track my progress. I've found the use of this type of self-accountability particularly useful when trying to establish a new routine. For instance, when I was working towards drinking eight to ten glasses of water per day, I used MyFitnesspal to alert me to drink water and as a way to track how many glasses I had consumed each day. Eventually, this became routine for me, and I no longer needed the reminder, but it was very helpful for the first month of trying to establish this new behavior.

All of the goals within your plan will require, at the very least, a form of self-accountability or boosted self-accountability in order to accomplish them. However, there is a good chance that you will identify one or more goal(s) within your plan that you could use a little outside help getting off the ground. In these instances, it would be helpful to consider incorporating extrinsic accountability. The most common form of extrinsic accountability is to utilize family and/or friends for support.

Family/Friends Accountability

For all of us, there are going to be goals that are particularly challenging to accomplish and that require a layer of accountability beyond ourselves. Calling on family and/or friends to provide this accountability can be extremely beneficial.

Take a moment and think about your day-to-day activities. In what ways are you already held accountable by your family and friends? For me, most of the things I do outside of the workplace include some accountability to my daughter and my wife. For instance, my daughter needs to be at daycare by 8:00 a.m. This deadline holds me accountable by making sure I complete my morning routine and leave the house by 7:30 each day. In the evening, if I want my wife to be able to have a few minutes to relax before bedtime, certain tasks need to be completed, dinner being made, dishes cleaned, dog walked, etc. It is important to me that my wife has some time to decompress, which holds me accountable for completing these tasks. As you can see, much of our accountability from friends and family is baked into our daily lives, often without us even thinking about it; however, when seeking accountability to accomplish goals outside of the status quo, it is important to set up structures to ensure that the accountability will have the intended impact. Here are some guidelines on how to make an effective accountability plan when utilizing family and friends.

Family

Let's start off by discussing who you should not seek accountability from. Right away, I would suggest ruling out your significant other or parents. The reason behind this is they are hardwired to love you unconditionally, and it often serves in their best interest to let you off the hook relatively easily. I certainly am not going to give my wife a hard time for skipping a workout if it means she is going to be upset with me or it is going to make her feel guilty about not following through on a commitment. I can just hear the conversation now . . .

Me: You had mentioned that you wanted me to remind you about your workout tonight. Is that something you still plan to do?

My wife: I know, but I am just too tired tonight.

Me: I'm sure you are, but you have been saying for a while that you want to get back to exercising regularly and that you wanted me to hold you accountable.

My wife: Are you saying that I'm lazy and out of shape?

Me: No, not at all. Forget it; let's just watch Netflix . . .

I know I'm not the only significant other that would quickly drop the role of accountability partner in order to maintain homeostasis within my relationship. For this reason, plan to avoid asking your partner to hold you accountable to your goals. Trust me; you'll both be happier for it. Likewise, a parent isn't a great choice to provide external accountability, but there are plenty of other family members that can fill this role.

Asking a sibling, cousin, aunt, or uncle to help hold you accountable to your goals can be a very effective way to increase your rate of success. Usually, there is the right level of closeness and trust built into these relationships to make them strong choices for accountability partners. However, these relationships are much different than that of a spouse or parent, which makes it easier for these people to be honest with you and to provide pushback without fear of damaging your relationship. This same type of dynamic usually exists with friendships as well.

Friends

We all have at least one friend that tells it how it is. I know most of mine certainly do, albeit some gentler than others. All of my close friends I've known since high school, some since kindergarten, which means these friends know me well. I mean, really know the fabric of who I am as a person. Due to this closeness, they are not afraid, nor would I be, to be completely honest with them. I'm sure as you're reading this, you are thinking of friendships you have that fit this same mold. These types of friends make for very effective accountability partners.

Friends are a great source of accountability because they are invested in your life, their opinions matter to you, and they can provide you with honest feedback without the limitations that are naturally built into the relationship you have with your spouse and parents. When thinking about what friends to choose, try to identify a friend who is likely to be able to connect with you about the incremental behavioral efforts you are making rather than someone who is more likely to give you praise for your innate abilities. This type of feedback is more likely to help lead you to better outcomes[1]. The friend you choose to help provide you with accountability doesn't have to be someone you've known since grade school, although it can be. It does have to be a friend that you trust and who knows you well enough to be able to understand when you need to be pushed and when you need an empathetic ear. If you don't think you have a friend that fits this mold, perhaps you should consider leveraging organized support.

Organized Support

Organized support comes in many different shapes and sizes. For our purposes, we'll discuss the two most prevalent forms of organized support, which are group support and professional support.

Group Support

Group support comes in several forms, but the two most utilized are a group of people who are working on the same type of behavior change and are interested in connecting about their common efforts or a group of people who want to actively participate in change together. If you are interested in connecting with people who are working on similar goals, you are in luck because virtually any goal you can think of has multiple online support groups that anyone with a device can access. These groups can be found through apps such as MyFitnesspal, social media platforms like Facebook, and support forums such as "3 Fat Chicks." These groups can certainly be used as a source of accountability and can also serve as a source of inspiration and education. Depending on your goals, you can also find in-person support groups that offer routine meetings. On the other hand, if you prefer to actively work on your goals with other people, you may be more inclined to join an activity-based support group.

Activity-based support groups or clubs are similar to traditional support groups, but rather than supporting each other purely through discussion, groups of people get together to work on their goals. The most common form of activity-based groups is focused on exercise. In nearly every community, there are groups of people meeting on a routine basis to exercise together. These groups could be focused on hiking, walking, jogging, or training for a specific goal, such as a triathlon. There is a group for just about every type and level of activity you can think of. Joining one of these groups can be a nice way to add an extra layer of outside accountability and meet new people who are working on similar goals. Although support groups can be an excellent form of accountability, some people prefer the guidance of a trained professional.

Professional Support

There are certainly instances where accountability provided by a trained professional is exactly what a person needs to get their goals off the ground. These professionals are able to provide someone with a high level of objective accountability because their sole focus is to help their client achieve their goals. Now, as a trained Wellcoaches Health Coach, I'm, of course, partial to seeking support from a certified health coach because of the training they receive specific to facilitating behavior change. However, depending on the type of goal you are working to achieve and the frequency of accountability you are looking for, there are numerous wellness professionals that you can enlist to provide you with guidance and accountability. These professionals include but are not limited to: mental health counselors, registered dieticians, personal trainers, and health care providers.

Building Accountability Into Your Goals

Now that you understand how building accountability into your plan will increase your rate of goal achievement and you have given thought to what form(s) of accountability will work best for you, it's time to build a system of accountability into your plan. To do this, please return to your planning template and assign an accountability plan to each of your three-month behavioral goals. As previously mentioned, each of your goals may require different levels and forms of accountability. For instance, the goals that are most challenging for you to accomplish will likely need a form of external accountability, while others will come easier to you and will only require self-accountability. Here is what Katy's plan looked like after she added in her accountability plans:

Behavioral Goals:

1. Perform at least 90 minutes of cardiovascular exercise 3 days/week.

Accountability Plan: Draw a stick figure on my calendar each day I go to the gym

Potential barriers:

Back-up plans:

Stage of change: Preparation

2.Track all of the food I eat 7 days a week using a digital app

Accountability Plan: Built-in accountability within the app

Potential barriers:

Back-up plans:

Stage of change: Preparation

3.Plan 3 meals that include lean protein, whole grains, and vegetables, each week before going to the grocery store

Accountability Plan: Record my meal plan in my planner

Potential barriers:

Back-up plans: Stage of change: Preparation

4.5 nights a week, eat a dinner consisting of a plate made up of ½ fruits/vegetables, ¼ protein, ¼ carbohydrate

Accountability Plan: Report back to Ryan on the balanced nature of my meals

Potential barriers:

Back-up plans:

Stage of change: Preparation

5.Perform 10-15 minutes of strength training at least twice a week

Accountability Plan: Check in with personal trainer at the gym

Potential barriers:

Back-up plans:

Stage of change: Contemplation

Katy: Unsurprisingly, accountability has been an integral part of my journey pretty much from Day 1 when I started drawing little stick figures on my calendar each day I managed to get out and go for a walk. This, and other forms of Boosted Self-Accountability served me for a long while. I implemented a rule wherein I could only listen to certain podcasts while I was walking and I held myself to that rule! I made it a goal to walk at least 10,000 steps a day and started writing the number of steps my pedometer recorded at the end of every day on my calendar. I made little challenges for myself like seeing how far I could walk and/or how fast I could get from Point A to Point B. For years, these forms of Boosted Self-Accountability were the sole forms of accountability I was interested in using. I felt intensely private about my health journey and did not want to expose my goals and/or my methods to anyone else's scrutiny and/or advice. I think after years of "free advice" I'd been given about my health, I learned to enjoy the work I was doing on my own and felt immensely proud of what I was able to achieve.

After awhile, I occasionally shared big milestones (e.g., when I made it to 100 consecutive weeks of walking!) with very close friends and family and I realize now this was my foray into friends/family accountability. Even so, it took me several years before I formally invited any close family/friends or professionals into an external accountability circle.

After all that time relying on Boosted Self-Accountability, I started to flounder a bit in my health journey. At that time, I had just finished an advanced degree and moved to Boston to work in a research lab. My weight was beginning to creep up after I'd lost 100 pounds and I started to panic that I couldn't maintain and/or lose any more weight. It was at this point that I was invited to meet with Ryan through my primary care physician. At first, I was not interested. I had relied on my own self-accountability up to that point and unfortunately, viewed it as a weakness to turn to an outside person for accountability. I now recognize how wrong-headed that thinking is. To ask for external support and accountability takes a huge amount of **courage**; it's not weakness. Even so, when Ryan and I first met, I felt equal parts pride for what I had accomplished on my own thus far but also shame for the progress I'd lost and feared I would continue to lose.

When I first started meeting with Ryan, I was not very skilled or graceful about having an outside source of accountability. I just wasn't. I saw him as more of an outside judger and less of a cheerleader encouraging me on. It took a few months for me to change my attitude toward him. We had an initial meeting and I disclosed some of the things I struggled with but also didn't yet feel comfortable fully opening up to him. In that first meeting, I was careful to highlight the things I'd done and the things that were going well and only glossed over the things I struggled with. We talked about some goals I had and agreed to follow-up in six weeks. To be honest, I kept Ryan (and my goals!) largely out of my mind until right before we were to have a phone call to chat. And then I would panic! It was not unlike the panic that anyone who has taken music lessons but fails to practice until just before their next lesson feels. Ugh, those initial conversations with Ryan felt so awkward as I rambled about my excuses for why I hadn't gotten to where I wanted to be with my half-hearted attempts to reach my goals. At some point, we agreed to do an in-person meeting instead of another phone call. That in-person meeting wasn't much different than the phone calls. It was just me rambling about why I hadn't achieved my goals and feeling so relieved when I could leave the office. In short, the outside accountability wasn't working for me (but nor was my self-accountability either). Something needed to change.

I don't remember who suggested it, but the question was raised that perhaps six weeks was too long to go between conversations. I decided to start emailing Ryan once a week to let him know how my week had gone in regard to the goals I had set. This was a game changer. Those weekly emails became an extremely important source of accountability for me in three ways. First, it forced me to consciously consider my goals every. Single. Week. I couldn't just ignore my six-week, twelve-week, and year-long goals because I was emailing Ryan every week! Those weekly emails kept my goals at the forefront of my mind and, after a few weeks, I started looking forward to reporting on all the progress I was making. You may find that weekly check-ins are too frequent for you (or maybe not frequent enough!). If you're finding that a professional accountability source is not working for you, it may be that the timing is not quite right. Make some adjustments and see if that helps.

Secondly, emailing was a really helpful medium for me to check in with Ryan (versus a phone call or an in-person visit). Each week (generally on Monday morning), I would sit down and, on my own, reflect on my progress toward my goals over the previous week. I found the process of writing out and articulating my thoughts to be highly therapeutic and helpful. I needed that private space and time to honestly sort out how I was doing – and that was really difficult for me to do in a live conversation on the phone or in-person. By taking the time to write an email, I was able to think through situations and articulate how they were or were not helping me in regard to my overall goals. Writing things out gave me insight about why particular situations went well and/or why others didn't go so well. These emails were usually not very long. I generally included a statement of how the week had gone overall (good, so-so, not so great) and then selected a couple of specific happenings or aha moments that happened over the week. After I'd been emailing for a few weeks, and after I had finally been willing to set a weight-loss goal, I started including a postscript with my weight for the week.

Thirdly, as a wellness coach, Ryan was quite skilled at being the right kind of accountability. He responded to my emails with encouragement and congratulations when things went well, but just as often he responded with further questions and/or things for me to consider in my own reflection. These were not pointed questions such as "Why don't you try XX?" or "How could you have gotten yourself into that situation?" or "Why do you keep struggling with this?" His thoughtful questions were usually along the lines of, "Have you considered . . . " or "What do you think might be a good next step?" His questions encouraged more of my own introspection which allowed me to step up my game. He was so good at this. If you are seeking a professional source of accountability, I would encourage you to find a source that supports you in doing the work and not someone who tries to do the work **for you** and/or someone who tells you what to do. Over time, I began to see Ryan as more of a mentor who was guiding me through a process than a person I was checking in with to make sure I was on track. This was the kind of outside accountability that worked well for me – but it took a few weeks and months to find that right balance of support. It might take you a bit of trial and error to figure out what works for you too.

After some time, I started intentionally seeking outside sources of accountability within my own circle of family and friends. This step, for some reason, was a scary one to me. Confiding my goals and health ambitions to those close to me meant that I had to risk vulnerability which is not always easy for me. I didn't really like people being all up in my business and I was worried people would bug me, judge me, or question my methods. Thankfully, a dear friend opened the door for me as she first confided some of **her** own health goals to me. I took a leap of faith and decided to open up to her about some of my own goals. How did this happen? Clearly we had a mutual trust in each other. She felt safe with me and I felt safe with her. For me, I found it helpful that we shared vulnerabilities – we both were taking a risk and we both had something to gain by confiding in each other. In that conversation, we decided to even set a goal together: to run a 5K. We regularly checked in with each other and, six months later, we ran that 5K. In time, I started including other people in my circle of accountability: family, friends, colleagues. I have learned the value of my tribe knowing my goals and what I am working on. When I'm open about my goals, they encourage me and, I have found, can better support me in my quest to reach my goals. For several years, I found it difficult to navigate mealtimes when I visited my parents' house. Although the food offerings were always delicious (not to mention comforting with that taste of home!), sometimes the ingredients used or the dishes selected were at odds with my eating plans. It became a source of anxiety and frustration as I would frequently overeat and/or consume food that would push me over my calorie budget. At some point, it occurred to me, I was only frustrated because I hadn't actually communicated to my parents what my eating goals were. By not including them in my accountability circle, they had no idea how to support my health goals. I felt like they were sabotaging my goals when, in reality, I had not shared with them what I needed! On one visit home, I explained how I liked to set up my dinner: I usually chose a protein of some kind, a couple of vegetables, and sometimes a starch. Imagine my surprise when, the very next night, my dad came in the house with tomatoes and a zucchini from his beautiful garden. He set the veggies on the table and then walked to the fridge declaring, "Now we need a protein!" That one conversation invited him into my accountability circle and he was more than delighted to support me and my goals. In the end, I have found that accountability is about trust and support. When I trust others with my goals and need for support, they often reciprocate and it strengthens our relationship, which is a pretty great outcome.

What's Next?

You are getting excitingly close to launching your weight-loss plan. In fact, by the end of the next chapter, you will have set it in motion! But before you launch, there are a few other important aspects of the plan you need to initiate: identifying potential barriers and creating back-up plans. In the next chapter, you'll add these final pieces to your planning template, which will be followed by the setting of two-week goals in order to launch your plan.

Chapter Twelve Key Takeaways:

- External accountability has been shown to increase the rate of goal achievement.

- Boosted self-accountability can be leveraged by verbalizing and writing down your goals, creating visual reminders, and by using technology.

- External accountability can be procured by enlisting the support of family, friends, groups of people, and professionals.

Chapter Twelve To-Do List:

Before reading Chapter Thirteen, please make sure that you have completed each of these actions and added them to your planning template:

- ✓ Decide what type of accountability you'll need in order to achieve each of your three-month goals.

- ✓ Add an accountability plan to each of your three-month goals.

Chapter 13

Launching Your Weight-Loss Plan

Step 5: Launch Your Weight-Loss Plan

When I was growing up, my family rarely went on extravagant vacations; however, we were always guaranteed a week-long vacation on Cape Cod every summer. We lived just ninety minutes from our rental house on the Cape, but like clockwork, each year, we'd hit enough traffic during our annual pilgrimage to ensure that the car ride lasted at least two and a half hours. Most years, my two younger sisters and I were stuffed in the back of a station wagon, along with all of the other "essentials" we'd need for the week (bikes, beach toys, baseball gloves, fishing poles, etc.), usually without air-conditioning. As you can imagine, after several hours in the car we were hot, sticky, and generally on each other's last nerve. But at the end of each ride, there was a moment that made all the aggravation worthwhile.

This moment would arrive once we got close enough to the beach to taste the sea salt and smell the tanginess of the fresh ocean air. These sensations would wash over my siblings and me and put us all at ease, as they signaled that we had made it and that a week's worth of family fun was in front of us. In regards to your weight-loss journey, you are on the verge of arriving at this moment. You have endured the long drive, the heat, and the bickering, and you are nearly ready to reap the benefits.

To review, at this point in your journey, you have created a planning template that includes; your values, your one-year wellness vision, your three-month goals, and your accountability plan. This means that the last steps you need to take in order to finalize and subsequently launch your plan are to identify potential barriers, set up a check-in schedule, and create two-week goals. After taking these last few steps, you will be ready to take sustainable action by launching your plan! So let's not waste another minute and get to work on identifying potential barriers and creating back-up plans. Get ready to smell that ocean air!

Identifying Potential Barriers

Our natural inclination as human beings is to start working on goals and then deal with barriers as they arise. Although being able to pivot and make adjustments on the fly are certainly important traits to have in order to successfully reach your goals, by pre-identifying likely barriers that could stand in the way of goal achievement, you will dramatically increase your chances of success. One of my favorite quotes is "forethought is the antidote to distraction," which is definitely applicable in this situation as a touch of upfront planning can save you from a boatload of frustration and wasted energy down the line.

In order to identify potential barriers, you'll need to draw on the knowledge you have accumulated from your past experiences. To access this knowledge, in order to predict potential barriers, look at each of your three-month goals individually, and predict what barrier(s) might pop-up that could throw you off course. Here are some examples of the most frequently cited barriers to common behavioral goals:

Goal	Common external barriers
Cardiovascular exercise	• Lack of time • Bad weather • Schedule constraints
Calorie tracking	• Going out to eat • Not knowing what a serving size is considered • Forgetting to track
Eating 5 servings of fruits and vegetables a day	• Not having access to fresh produce • Not being able to measure a serving • Produce spoiling in between trips to the grocery store

Now is a good time to review each one of your three-month behavioral goals and brainstorm potential barriers that could arise and impede your progress. Please add these potential barriers to your planning template. Now that you have identified potential barriers,

I'll ask you to turn your attention towards addressing these barriers before they arise by creating backup plans.

Backup Planning

There is no mystery when it comes to creating backup plans. What you'll need to do is examine the potential barriers you came up with for each of your goals and create plans that you'll use if/when these barriers arise. Of course, it is impossible to plan for every potential barrier, but the idea is to identify the barriers that you are likely to encounter and create a backup plan in case they arise. To get a sense of what these plans might entail, I've added a backup plan for each potential barrier to the list that I shared with you in the previous section:

Goal	Common external barriers	Backup plans
Cardiovascular exercise	Lack of time	Exercise first thing in the morning so that I always have time built into my day
	Bad weather	Download group exercise classes that I can utilize if the weather doesn't allow for outdoor exercise

	Schedule constraints	Walk for 15 minutes during my lunch break and 15 minutes in the evening, rather than for 30 minutes at a time
Calorie tracking	Going out to eat	Look up the calories in the food I want to eat before leaving the house
	Not knowing a serving size	Use a cheat sheet to determine common servings sizes for foods
	Forgetting to track	Use a tracking app and set reminders to alert me to log my calories around mealtimes
Eating 5 servings of fruits and vegetables a day	Not having access to fresh produce during the day	Purchase portable produce that I can bring with me to work (bananas, apples, carrot sticks)
	Not being able to measure a serving	Look up serving-size estimates for raw and cooked produce
	Produce spoiling in between trips to the grocery store	Purchase frozen and shelf-stable produce to keep at home and at work

Before adding your own backup plans to your planning template, please take a look at the potential barriers and backup plans that Katy created within her plan:

Behavioral Goals:

1.Perform at least 90 minutes of cardiovascular exercise 3 days/week.

Accountability Plan: Draw a stick figure on my calendar each day I go to the gym

Potential barriers: Lack of time, finding the time to get to the gym

Back-up plans: Schedule it in my planner

Stage of change: Preparation

2.Track all of the food I eat 7 days a week using a digital app

Accountability Plan: Built-in accountability within the app

Potential barriers: Lack of habit

Back-up plans: Plan to log food during my commute on the train

Stage of change: Preparation

3.Plan 3 meals that include lean protein, whole grains, and vegetables, each week before going to the grocery store

Accountability Plan: Record my meal plan in my planner

Potential barriers: Lack of planning

Back-up plans: Choose a day/time of the week (Saturday morning) to make a plan before I go shopping

Stage of change: Preparation

4.5 nights a week, eat a dinner consisting of a plate made up of ½ fruits/vegetables, ¼ protein, ¼ carbohydrate

Accountability Plan: Report back to Ryan on the balanced nature of my meals

Potential barriers: Lack of knowledge on foods that have the targeted macronutrients

Back-up plans: Create a list of healthy foods to pick from

Stage of change: Preparation

5. Perform 10-15 minutes of strength training at least twice a week

Accountability Plan: Check in with personal trainer at the gym

Potential barriers: Lack of knowledge of exercises to do and/or how to work the weight machines at the gym

Back-up plans: Review YouTube videos to learn exercises; have a session with personal trainer

Stage of change: Contemplation

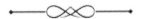

Katy: Anticipating and planning for barriers has been a crucial part of the success of my journey. I wish I were better at spotting those barriers before they cause me to stumble in my journey but often, I don't identify them until they have tripped me up a few times. Here are a few barriers that, over the years, I have identified and now actively create backup plans to intercept the barrier before it even starts:

Barrier #1: Getting derailed in my exercise plans when I go out of town and visit friends or family

Backup plan: I have learned how to be largely successful in my daily routine in my own life. This becomes much more of a challenge when I'm visiting family or friends and have less control over my daily schedule, less control over the food available, and less available access to my typical exercise options like the gym. It was especially difficult because for many years, I lived hundreds of miles away from my family. We are very close-knit and so going to visit was a special time when we'd try to eke out all the visiting time we could manage. I used to feel guilty about leaving for an hour to go for a walk/jog to exercise and "wasting" precious time we could have spent together. Fortunately, I've managed the exercise conundrum by, over the years, creating an expectation that I will exercise every morning when I'm visiting. At first, my family thought it was odd and would regularly comment about my odd insistence to go on a walk every morning. I've been doing this consistently for so many years now, everyone in my extended family now knows that I will be heading out on a walk/jog in the morning and no one even questions it anymore. To my utter delight, now when I visit, family members will ask **me**, "Katy, are you walking in the morning? Can I come with you?" It's been the most gratifying experience to be playing a small part in members of my family adopting healthy routines like regularly going for walks in the morning. Now it's rare for me to **not** have someone with me on those walks.

Barrier #2: Getting derailed on my eating plans when I travel

Backup Plan: Over the years, I have adopted several strategies that help keep me on track with my eating habits when I travel. I travel a fair amount for my job and, in the past, I tended to rely on airport kiosks, corner markets, and business lunches/dinners as my food plan. Not only did this present a problem for my wellness vision, it was downright expensive! Food-wise, I found that it was hard to control the food I had access to, and it was very difficult to find consistently nutritionally-balanced options. What to do? I have used the following ways to address these barriers:

1. Before the trip, I pre-package snacks I am willing to eat (single servings of nuts, carrot sticks, cheese sticks, jerky) and keep those in my bag at all times. Whenever I feel hungry, I know these are the snacks I can reach for without worry about derailing my eating goals.

2. If it's a multiday trip, I try to find a grocery store after I arrive and stock my hotel refrigerator with fresh fruits/veggies that are

easy to consume like pre-cut vegetables and hummus, boxed salads, etc. I also look for easy protein options like hard-boiled eggs, nuts, or jerky with no added sugar to help with satiety.

3. When I need to eat out for business purposes, I steer myself to salads and fresh vegetable options and away from heavy dishes with lots of starches and sauces. I have learned that my stomach will feel much more settled with the fresh vegetable options. The heavy food just doesn't sit well anymore and it is just plain no fun to travel when your gut feels unhappy.

Barrier #3: How to handle unanticipated social events (birthday parties, social get-togethers) where I am not in control of the food menu and/or it's potluck style

Backup plan: I've handled this situation in a couple of ways. One strategy is to make sure that I eat a snack before the event so that I'm not starving. If I go to an event very hungry, I am bound to eat more food than I need for my eating plan. A second strategy is to do a walkthrough at the food table and decide ahead of time what I'm going to select rather than decide as I go. This seems like a small distinction but it has helped me a lot. When I'm deciding what food to select as I'm going, I'm much more likely to put much more food on my plate because I don't want to miss out on anything. A related strategy is to load my plate with mostly greens/salad which makes the remaining part of the plate visibly smaller and thus, I dish up less food.

Barrier #4: The holidays

Backup Plan: Here's an excerpt from an email I sent to Ryan in early December 2015 as I was preparing for the holiday season:

"The next three weeks are arguably the most difficult for me food-wise, out of the whole year. This week alone, I will have only one dinner at home. There are unstructured gatherings, dinners out, holiday treats EVERYwhere, and then I head out to visit my family next week. I think, for my benefit, I just want to review the strategies that have worked in the past so I can feel confident in my game plan.

A few things that work well:

- ✓ Use my travel strategies (pack individual portion sizes of good snacks and veggies, etc)

- ✓ For meals out: do your best to select food that is close to what you would normally eat at home: a lean protein, lots of veggies, avoid cheeses/creamy sauces

- ✓ Pack gum. Always have gum with you. :-)

- ✓ Plan ahead for treats. Consider the treats you think you might want to eat and decide when you're going to have them.

- ✓ Remember that "social pressure to eat this" is not a good reason to eat something. Do you want to eat the food? Then great. If you're feeling obligated to eat the food, reconsider.

- ✓ Log what you eat. Always!

✓ The kitchen is closed after 8 pm. Remember, nothing good comes from eating after 8 pm. Like, ever.

✓ Get in your exercise - whatever it takes."

It's been five years since I wrote that email and these are still the strategies I try to implement when December rolls around.

These are just a few barriers I've encountered in my own experience and have worked to strategically overcome. I'm not perfect at implementing these strategies, but I've come a long way over the years. You may look at my list of barriers and feel like they wouldn't really present as barriers to you. That's okay! Your barriers may look quite different from mine. Anything that keeps you from meeting your goals and/or keeping to your wellness vision is a barrier. You will likely need to use trial and error to find the strategies that make **your** back-up plans successful. But with self-reflection and trying to implement different strategies, you will find what works for you!

As you can see, Katy was able to get out in front of barriers that, if unplanned for, would have caused her to be thrown off course from reaching her goals. In order to do the same, please add your own backup plans to your planning template before moving on to set your two-week goals.

Setting Two-Week Goals

One of the final steps you need to take before putting your plan into action is to set two-week goals. This two-week time span has been selected because it is a long enough sample size to get a clear sense of how you are progressing with your goals but short enough so that there is still a sense of urgency to complete your goals.

Your two-week goals should be written in support of your three-month goals and should be set within your current stage of change. To create your two-week goals, please follow these steps:

1. Pick one of the behavioral three-month goals that you are ready to get moving on.

2. Determine what stage of change you are in currently in regards to that goal.

3. Create a S.M.A.R.T. goal that allows you to take a step forward within the appropriate stage of change. The goal you create should feel like an action you are confident in accomplishing within the next two weeks.

4. Examine the potential barriers you listed related to the goal you decide to work on and set a backup plan, if necessary.

5. Repeat this process until you have created at least two but no more than three two-week goals.

Here is what Katy's first set of two-week goals looked like:

Behavioral Goals:

1.Run/walk outside for at least 30 minutes on Tuesday and Thursday morning before work

Stage of change: Action

Potential barriers: Rainy weather

Back-up plans: Run/walk on the treadmill after work on Tuesday and Thursday

2.Read at least one review article on Saturday about food tracking apps and pick one to download.

Stage of change: Preparation

Potential barriers: Getting busy and forgetting to read the article

Back-up plans: Block time in my Outlook calendar to read the article on Monday morning

Once you have created your two-week goals, you'll need to create a check-in plan so that you can measure your progress and set new goals that will keep you moving toward achieving your three-month goals every two weeks.

Creating a Check-In Plan

Last but not least, take the time to create a check-in plan that will require you to measure the progress you've made on your goals every two weeks. You should do this by scheduling time on your calendar to review your two-week goals and to set new two-week goals. This check-in should be self-managed but can include an accountability partner if you have integrated one as part of your plan.

During your two-weeks goal check-in time, you should follow these steps when assessing your progress:

1. Look at each of your two-week goals and assign a "percent complete" to each goal on a scale of 0 to 100 percent

2. If you scored 100 percent complete on the goal, ask yourself: What went right, and what do I need to continue to do to make sure that I stay on track?

3. If you scored less than 100 percent on the goal, ask yourself: What didn't go as planned, and what adjustments do I need to make in order to reach this goal?

4. Once you have reviewed each two-week goal, check in on your three-month goals by asking yourself the following questions:

    a. What type of progress am I making toward my outcome goal?

    b. Do I need to update my stage of change in any of these goals?

    c. What two-week goals do I need to set today in order to move closer toward achieving my three-month goals?

5. Finally, based on the answers to these questions, set new two-week goals, and schedule a new time to check in with yourself.

Keeping Katy's example in mind, return to your planning template and add two to three, two-week goals, and a check-in plan to your weight-loss template. Once you have done this, you are ready to launch your plan!

Launching Your Plan

You have reached the most crucial part of this book. Leading up to this section, you have acquired the knowledge necessary to fully understand exactly what you need to do to make sustainable behavior changes in order to achieve and maintain your ideal weight. Additionally, you have created a bulletproof plan that will allow you to operationalize this knowledge, which now lives on your completed weight-loss plan template. However, knowledge acquisition and planning will not change your life but applying this knowledge through the execution of the plan you created *will* change your life. The question becomes, are you ready and willing to take action?

For most people, their first action after finishing a book is to start another book. If your next action after finishing this book is to read another book, then you are not going to lose a single pound. Your next action after finishing this book needs to be the execution of the plan you've created. In fact, Katy and I believe so strongly about the need for you to act that we are calling for you to launch your plan by participating in the Weight Lost 12-Week Challenge.

Weight Lost 12-Week Challenge

The Weight Lost 12-Week Challenge is a call to action that involves you putting the amazing plan that you've created, along with all of the knowledge you acquired during the course of reading this book, into motion. If you accept this challenge, launch your plan by executing your first two-week goals, utilizing your check-in plan, setting new two-week goals, and repeating this process six times over the next twelve weeks. Once you have completed the Weight Lost 12-Week Challenge, visit www.weightlostacademy.com to share your story! We'd love to hear about your successes and help to support you if you've run into challenges along the way. Also, feel free to share the progress you are making and gain support along the way by joining the WeightLost Facebook group. This is a great way to stay connected with Katy and me and other like-minded people who are executing their own Weight-Lost plan.

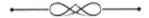

Katy: Launching your plan really **is** the exciting part. It's the action you've been waiting for, and now it's time to really get to work. By breaking your goals into incremental two-week goals, that will help things feel much more manageable. My advice is to reflect on your three-month goals but keep your focus on what you need to do for the next two weeks. It's easy for me to get overwhelmed thinking about all that I need to accomplish in three months, but a two-week time frame feels much more manageable. True confession: I sometimes even break it down into a week at a time. Because it's so important for my goals to feel achievable, I need to frame them in timelines and terms that feel achievable. Checking in with your accountability source (whether that's your own reflection, a trusted friend, a family member, or our online community) regularly will not only keep you motivated to stay on track, you'll find others who are there to support you in your bid for your own success. It is a beautiful thing to have a support network who is cheering you on, providing you a sounding board when you are overwhelmed or need help problem-solving challenging situations, and who ultimately believes that it is YOU that has the power to change your life. Because it's true. Your success is in your control, and it's time to launch!

What's Next?

After accepting the Weight Lost 12-Week Challenge, I know you will be excited to hit the ground running. However, before jumping at full speed, it's important to pause to think about how you plan to keep your reflective and goal-setting juices flowing after you've achieved your initial three-month goals.

Far too often, people start out of the gate with great focus and determination but seem to lose this momentum or become distracted as they attempt to move toward their ideal wellness vision. To ensure that the behavior changes you make are sustainable and that you reach your one-year vision, you'll need to put a plan in place that includes the setting of new goals every three months, the incremental celebration of accomplishments, and continuous learning. We'll cover these topics and more in the final chapter.

Chapter Thirteen Key Takeaways:

- Preemptively identifying potential barriers that could derail goal achievement and creating backup plans to move past these barriers will increase your rate of success.

- Setting two-week goals will allow you enough time to make progress on your goals but not so much time that you lose your sense of urgency.

- Creating a check-in plan for yourself will ensure that you stay on track toward reaching your three-month goals.

- Launching your plan by accepting the Weight Lost 12-Week Challenge is the first step toward achieving your ideal wellness vision and to changing your life.

Chapter Thirteen To-Do List:

Before reading Chapter Thirteen, please make sure that you have completed each of these actions and added them to your planning template:

- ✓ Identify potential barriers for each of your three-month goals.

- ✓ Identify backup plans for each of your three-month goals.

- ✓ Create your first set of two-week goals.

Launch your plan by accepting the Weight Lost 12-Week Challenge

Chapter 14

Maintaining Momentum

Several mornings each week, my boxer, Lucy, and I go for a long run. I like to use the app *Runkeeper* to track my pace and measure my progress over time. What I've found through tracking my runs is that each follows a very similar pattern. I start out of the gates running fast but then after a few minutes, reality kicks in. I can feel the heaviness of my legs and the fatigue from perhaps not sleeping great the night before, and as a result, my pace lessens. But then, about a third of the way into my run, I regain my momentum and end up finishing strong. In many ways, this is what your weight-loss journey is going to feel like.

Of the hundreds of patients I've worked with on weight loss, 90 percent fell into the same pattern of behavior change. They start out of the gates strong and lose a great deal of weight in months one to six. This strong start is often followed by a dip in energy and/or focus (usually because their plan is working so well). This is where the rubber meets the road. Some people will end their weight-loss journey right here, happy to have lost a significant amount of weight. However, others will continue to push forward by making goal setting and self-reflection part of their lifestyle. These are the people who not only go on to achieve their one-year wellness vision but create a new vision for themselves each year and end up leading a lifestyle and achieving a weight that they didn't even know was possible. Do you want to be this person? If so, the information provided in this chapter will be of great interest to you.

There are three factors that are of tremendous importance when considering how to reach your one-year wellness vision and beyond. These determinants are continuous goal setting and self-reflection, celebrating your accomplishments, and continuous growth. Let's look at each of these facets individually to better understand their importance.

Continuous Goal Setting and Self-Reflection

Accepting the Weight Lost 12-Week Challenge and following through on your first set of goals is a BIG deal. Proving that you can execute and adjust your personal weight-loss plan in order to achieve your outcome goal over a three-month period is certainly something to be proud of. However, achieving your first set of goals is really just the beginning, as what you are really interested in accomplishing is achieving your one-year vision. To do this, you'll need to implement a process of continuous goal setting and self-reflection. There are many ways to do this, but I'll share with you the structure of a three-month cycle that has worked for hundreds of my patients.

Working toward your one-year vision is an exciting process; however, it can be easy to lose focus on your goals over the course of a year, especially with everything else going on in your life. Therefore, it is important that you reflect on the progress you are making toward your one-year vision every three months and follow up this reflection by setting new three-month goals.

At the conclusion of every three-month period, you should review the progress you have made towards your three-month goals and assign yourself a "percent complete" for each goal. If you have been setting two-week goals all along, there should be no surprises during your three-month check-in. Before setting new three-month goals, you should take a moment to reflect on your one-year vision by asking yourself these questions:

- Is this still how you would like to see yourself and/or your life?

- Does this vision still excite you?

- Would reaching this vision still be meaningful to you?

- If the answers to any of these questions are "no," consider revising it before setting new three month goals.

Once you have achieved your one-year wellness vision, even if it was achieved quicker than anticipated (don't be surprised if you reach your original vision in just six months), it is time to dream up a new one-year wellness vision for yourself or set maintenance goals. But before examining what steps to take in order to maintain your efforts, let's take a moment to talk about a very important component of sustaining long-term success, which is often overlooked – celebrating your accomplishments.

Celebrating Accomplishments

By reading this book and creating your own weight-loss plan, you are well on your way to making sustainable behavior changes, which will allow you to permanently say goodbye to unwanted pounds. However, it would be deceiving to tell you that your plan will lead you to your ideal wellness vision in a linear fashion. For a very small percentage of you, making a b-line that leads directly to your ideal wellness vision might be a reality; however, for most people, the path to sustainable change is complicated with pauses in forward progress, unforeseen roadblocks, and even periods of regression. Without taking time to celebrate incremental progress, these totally normal bumps in the road on your way toward your ideal wellness vision will become understandably frustrating. However, celebrating incremental progress points on your way will make these temporary setbacks feel much more tolerable.

Taking time to celebrate each success you have, whether it be big or small, is an important way to reinforce your "I can do this" mentality and will help you to maintain your focus on your way to achieving your ideal wellness vision. You'll need to take just two steps to set up your incremental celebrations: first, decide which incremental achievements you'll celebrate, we'll call these "celebration points," and second, decide how you'll celebrate.

Celebration Points

To identify celebration points, decide what incremental markers, once achieved, will be meaningful to you. For instance, if your three-month goal is to lose 12 pounds, then you could make losing 6 pounds (halfway to your goal) a celebration point. Or if your goal is to drink eight glasses of water a day, but you are starting at just two glasses per day, make drinking four glasses a day a celebration point. Let's look at Katy's one-year ideal wellness vision and three-month goals in order to identify what her celebration points could have been:

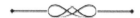

Katy: A few months after I met Ryan, I set my first weight loss goal: I wanted to weigh less than 200 pounds. I had not been in the 100's since I was a young teenager, and I finally felt like maybe it could be within reach. At the time, I weighed 225 pounds. The lowest I had weighed in adulthood was 215 pounds, so I decided that my first celebration point would be when I got below 215 pounds. And I celebrated! It felt good to have achieved a weight I'd never seen in my adult life! How did I celebrate? I remember sending an excited email to Ryan, letting him know and that felt enough for me. After several months of hard work and effort, my weight fluctuating up and down in 2–3 pound increments, I finally got within reach of 200 pounds. I floated just above 200 pounds for a few painstaking weeks. It was **so** frustrating! I'd get within reach of 199 pounds and then float back up a couple of pounds. Eventually, one glorious morning, I saw 199 on the scale as I stepped on it. I'm not sure I can adequately describe the feeling I had when I reached this momentous milestone. Did I celebrate? Of course I did! I took a picture of the number on the scale and sent it to Ryan, to my sister, and to a close friend. I excitedly announced it to my roommate. The support I felt from my tribe was phenomenal. The next milestone I wanted to celebrate was 188 pounds. Why? Because that number was going to represent me having lost 40 percent of my body weight from my peak weight of 315 pounds. My next milestone? 185.5 pounds. Why would I have a milestone only 2.5 pounds below my previous milestone? I had realized that when I reached 185.5 pounds, I would officially be classified as "Overweight" on the BMI, instead of "Obese." These were milestones that nobody else figured out for me – they were important just to **me**. And how did I celebrate? I sent Ryan an email in all caps that read "RYAN! I'M OVERWEIGHT!!!" I was never more proud to proclaim I was overweight.

I have had other notable celebration points that have not necessarily been connected to my weight. These have usually involved achieving a challenging physical feat or overcoming a particular fear. For example, I celebrated the day that I ran a mile in under eleven minutes (which was a huge feat for me!); I celebrated when I completed a fifteen-mile hike in one day; I celebrated when I completed an eighty-mile bike ride; I celebrated when I was able to hold a plank for ninety seconds. I celebrated when I wore a bathing suit without a shirt on; I celebrated when I wore a beautiful dress with confidence; I celebrated when I set and achieved a fitness goal with a friend. In each of these cases, I chose to celebrate achieving something that was either physically or mentally challenging.

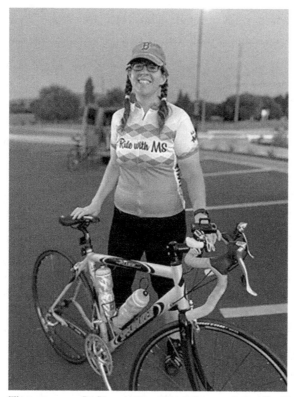

(This past summer, I celebrated biking 150+ miles over a 2-day bike ride with pizza and a good long nap!)

Importantly, I worked hard to avoid celebrating by taking a break from exercise or eating copious amounts of food that weren't part of my eating plan. I have tried to identify ways to celebrate that don't undo all the progress I've made! I've celebrated by traveling to a new place; I've celebrated by going ziplining (something I was unable to do when I was heavier); I've celebrated by buying a new piece of hiking or camping gear I've been wanting; and yes, I've celebrated by getting a really good burger to eat after a 3-day backpacking trip where I hiked over 25 miles. My celebrations are much more supportive of my overall goals when I plan ahead for them. I would encourage you to identify those things that align with your overall wellness vision.

Celebrating Incremental Progress

Once you have decided on your celebration points, it's time to party! Well, I guess you could throw a party when you reach each celebration point, but celebrating doesn't have to involve throwing a party or some other grand gesture. However, your celebration, whether big or small, should mark the moment in your mind and should also be meaningful to you. Here are a few tips on how to celebrate your achievements in a meaningful way:

- Do:
  - Connect your celebration to your values. For instance, as you'll recall, what I value the most is family, so a meaningful celebration for me might be to go on a hike with my wife and daughter or to take my daughter and my dad to a baseball game.

  - Connect the celebration to your goals. An example of this might be to treat yourself to a three-month subscription to *Spotify* so you can listen to it while you walk or to sign up for a meal kit delivery service like *Blue Apron*.

- Don't:
  - Celebrate by splurging on something that is outside of your value set or is in conflict with your goals. This

type of celebration is often a trip to a fast-food restaurant or a "cheat day" of eating unhealthy foods.

o   Make the celebration a huge lift. The last thing you want to do is do more work for yourself, so don't plan a celebration that will add stress to your life. Sometimes, just a thirty-minute bubble bath without interruptions is the best way to celebrate.

Whatever celebrations you come up with, make sure you follow through on them. Following through on your celebrations is just as important as following through with your goals. Yes, you want to stay driven and focused on achieving your ideal wellness vision, but you also want to enjoy the journey. In addition to using celebrations to keep your plan exciting and fresh, investing in continuous learning and personal growth can also help to keep the fire within you burning strong.

Continuing to Learn and Challenge Yourself

I have no doubt that if you follow the strategies outlined in this book that you will reach all of your goals and attain your ideal wellness vision. However, the downside of reaching your goals is that you can become complacent, which can be a slippery slope leading back into old, unwanted habits. The good news is that there are two strategies that you can use to avoid complacency: maintenance goal setting and continuous growth.

Maintenance goal setting is a straightforward concept: identify the behaviors that you need to continue to perform in order to maintain your ideal wellness vision. By the time you have achieved your wellness vision, you'll most likely have a very good handle on the behaviors that are most crucial for you to continue with in order to maintain the weight loss you have achieved. However, if you aren't sure about what maintenance goals you should set for yourself, here are some of the most common maintenance goals people set for themselves in order to maintain their weight loss:

Maintenance Goal	Recommendation
Weighing themselves on a regular basis	Weigh yourself once a week
Performing regular exercise	Perform 150 minutes of moderate or 75 minutes of vigorous cardiovascular exercise and perform at least two days of strength training a week
Making healthy food choices	Eat at least 5 servings of fruits and vegetables a day, eat at least 25 grams of fiber each day, drink at least 8 glasses of water a day

Setting maintenance goals for yourself is a must for anyone who wants to say goodbye forever to the pounds they worked so hard to lose. Another important component of a successful weight-loss maintenance plan is to keep challenging yourself through continuous growth.

Continuous Growth

Through designing your own weight-loss plan that includes sustainable behavioral changes, you are primed to achieve your one-year wellness vision and maintain this vision well into the future. However, as we know, our lifestyle is an ever-changing entity that will demand that our habits evolve alongside it. No matter how ingrained our healthy habits are in our lives, we will be forced to make changes to our routines when major life events occur.

Significant life events like a new job, a new relationship, moving to a new home, or the birth of a child will usually result in a change in routine. But what shouldn't change are your personal values. As I've previously mentioned, one of my personal values is my health. One way I've always upheld this value is by exercising consistently. As a single man in my twenties, my routine was to spend an hour or more at the gym six days a week performing strength training and cardiovascular exercise. Heck, I would even play a little basketball after my workout if I felt like it! However, now, as a married man with a daughter and a dog, my lifestyle no longer supports this type of exercise routine, which has required that my habits evolve.

In order to figure out how to continue to exercise on a regular basis within the structure of my new lifestyle, I needed to figure out how to adjust my habits. This required me to do some reading and conduct other research so that I could figure out how to implement an at-home exercise routine that allowed me to continue to perform regular cardiovascular exercise and strength training while balancing my other responsibilities. It is inevitable that sometime in the future, you too will be faced with similar lifestyle changes that will call on you to continue to learn and grow so that you can figure out how to adapt your habits while continuing to uphold your personal values in order to pursue/sustain your ideal wellness vision.

Now, this adaption can go the other way as well. You may move to a warmer climate that allows you to start exercising outside more often, or your kids might go off to college, which gives you more time to experiment with cooking new recipes. Either way, changes in your lifestyle will provide opportunities for you to explore new ways of supporting your wellness vision. My hope for you is that you embrace these opportunities and enjoy the process of continuous growth. There will certainly be many different avenues for you to continue your weight loss and maintenance journey, and I encourage you to explore them all. I'd also encourage you to stay connected with Katy and me so that we can continue to support your efforts.

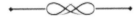

Katy: I cannot say enough about the importance of staying on a maintenance plan that ensures that your daily behaviors continue to align with your personal values. As Ryan points out, life has its natural ebbs and flows that come with major life events or subtle lifestyle changes. One of my core values is to ensure that I am always healthy enough to get outside and enjoy the great outdoors via camping, hiking, and exploring. Because this is a core value, I regularly incorporate plans for outdoor adventures (day trips, weekend trips, etc.) so that I am motivated to maintain my physical condition and stamina to actively participate in these activities. My plan is to just keep assuming that I can and will participate in these outdoor adventures. With that mindset, it is easy to continue to feel motivated to exercise regularly, eat well, and make sure my body stays healthy for such adventuring. What core values do you have? What is your vision for your wellness for the next three months? Six months? A year? Beyond? I am living proof that the key to achieving that vision is your own desire to do so. By using the principles in this book, you'll be able to articulate your vision, implement a scientifically-based plan, create a backup plan to preemptively attack barriers that may arise, and ultimately find the success you seek. You can do it! I know you can!

Staying Connected and Continuing to Learn

I certainly believe that by reading this book, you have the information and structure you need to achieve your ideal weight and wellness vision. But I also understand that people learn in different ways and benefit from different forms of support. For these reasons, we have developed several resources for you to use in order to continue learning and to gain future support:

Weight Lost Academy- www.weightlostacdemy.com

*Weight Lost Blog-*https://weightlostacademy.com/blog/

Email- weightlostacademy@gmail.com

We look forward to continuing to support you as you work toward your ideal weight and wellness vision and to hearing your success story!

Chapter Fourteen Key Takeaways:

- Establishing a process for regular self-reflection and goal setting will help you achieve your ideal one-year wellness vision.

- Celebrating incremental accomplishments will help to keep you motivated and excited about achieving your goals.

- Setting maintenance goals and continuing to learn about healthy lifestyle habits will help you achieve and sustain your ideal weight.

Chapter Fourteen To-Do List:

✓ Establish a schedule for reflecting on your progress and setting new goals every three months.

✓ Create incremental celebration points.

✓ Set maintenance goals once you have achieved your ideal weight.

✓ Stay connected with Ryan and Katy in order to continue to learn, gain support, and to share your success story.

Urgent Plea

Thank You For Reading Our Book!

We really appreciate all of your feedback, and love hearing what you have to say.

We need your input to make the next version of this book and our future books better.

Please leave us a helpful review on Amazon letting us know what you thought of the book.

Thank you,

Ryan and Katy

End Notes

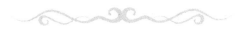

Introduction

1. Steeves, J. A., Liu, B., Willis, G., Lee, R., & Smith, A. W, "Physicians' Personal Beliefs About Weight-related Care and Their Associations with Care Delivery: the US National Survey of Energy Balance Related Care among Primary Care Physicians," Obesity Research & Clinical Practice, 9(3) (2015): 243-255.

2. Locke, E. A., "Toward a Theory of Task Motivation and Incentives," Organizational Behavior and Human Performance, 3(2) (1968): 157-189.

3. Locke, E. A., and Latham, G. P., "Building a Practically Useful Theory of Goal Setting and Task Motivation: A 35-Year Odyssey," American Psychologist, 57(9) (2002): 705.

4. Sherman, R. P., Petersen, R., Guarino, A. J., and Crocker, J. B, "Primary Care–Based Health Coaching Intervention for Weight Loss in Overweight/Obese Adults: A 2-Year Experience," American Journal of Lifestyle Medicine, 13(4) (2019): 405-413.

Chapter Two

1. Seligman, M. E., and Csikszentmihalyi, M., Positive psychology: An introduction. In Flow and the Foundations of Positive Psychology (Springer, Dordrecht, 2014), 279-298.

Chapter Three

1. Ranganathan, V. K., Siemionow, V., Liu, J. Z., Sahgal, V., and Yue, G. H.,"From Mental Power to Muscle Power—Gaining Strength by Using the Mind," Neuropsychologia, 42(7) (2004): 944-956.

2. Clark, B. C., Mahato, N. K., Nakazawa, M., Law, T. D., and Thomas, J. S., "The Power of the Mind: the Cortex as a Critical Determinant of Muscle Strength/Weakness," Journal of Neurophysiology, 112(12) (2014): 3219-3226.

Chapter Four

1. Wishnofsky, M., "Caloric Equivalents of Gained or Lost Weight," Journal of the American Medical Association, 173(1) (1960): 85-85.

2. Fothergill, E., Guo, J., Howard, L., Kerns, J. C., Knuth, N. D., Brychta, R., ... and Hall, K. D., "Persistent Metabolic Adaptation 6 Years After "The Biggest Loser" Competition," Obesity, 24(8) (2016): 1612-1619.

3. Benton, D., and Young, H. A., "Reducing Calorie Intake May Not Help You Lose Body Weight," Perspectives on Psychological Science, (2017).

Chapter Five

1. Rolls, B. J., Drewnowski, A., and Ledikwe, J. H., "Changing the Energy Density of the Diet as a Strategy for Weight Management," Journal of the American Dietetic Association, 105(5) (2005): 98-103.

2. Chambers, L., McCrickerd, K., and Yeomans, M. R., "Optimizing Foods for Satiety," Trends in Food Science & Technology, 41(2) (2015): 149-160.

3. C.S. Mott Children's Hospital. Fiber in Foods Chart. Michigan Medicine.   Retrieved   from: https://www.med.umich.edu/mott/pdf/mott-fiber-chart.pdf

4. Muckelbauer, R., Sarganas, G., Grüneis, A., and Müller-Nordhorn, J., "Association Between Water Consumption and Body Weight Outcomes: a Systematic Review," The American Journal of Clinical Nutrition, 98(2) (2013): 282-299.

5. Parretti, H. M., Aveyard, P., Blannin, A., Clifford, S. J., Coleman, S. J., Roalfe, A., and Daley, A. J., "Efficacy of Water Preloading Before Main Meals as a Strategy for Weight Loss in Primary Care Patients with Obesity," RCT. Obesity, 23(9) (2015): 1785-1791.

6. Dennis, E. A., Dengo, A. L., Comber, D. L., Flack, K. D., Savla, J., Davy, K. P., and Davy, B. M., "Water Consumption Increases Weight Loss During a Hypocaloric Diet Intervention in Middle-Aged and Older Adults," Obesity, 18(2) (2010): 300-307.

7. Boschmann, M., Steiniger, J., Hille, U., Tank, J., Adams, F., Sharma, A. M., ... and Jordan, J., "Water-Induced Thermogenesis,"The Journal of Clinical Endocrinology & Metabolism, 88(12) (2003): 6015-6019.

8. Boschmann, M., Steiniger, J., Franke, G., Birkenfeld, A. L., Luft, F. C., & Jordan, J., "Water Drinking Induces Thermogenesis Through Osmosensitive Mechanisms," The Journal of Clinical Endocrinology & Metabolism, 92(8) (2007): 3334-3337.

9. Stookey, J. D., Constant, F., Popkin, B. M., and Gardner, C. D., "Drinking Water is Associated with Weight Loss in Overweight Dieting Women Independent of Diet and Activity," Obesity, 16(11) (2008): 2481-2488.

10. Blom, W. A., Lluch, A., Stafleu, A., Vinoy, S., Holst, J. J., Schaafsma, G., and Hendriks, H. F., "Effect of a High-Protein Breakfast on the Postprandial Ghrelin Response," The American Journal of Clinical Nutrition, 83(2) (2006): 211-220.

11. Batterham, R. L., Heffron, H., Kapoor, S., Chivers, J. E., Chandarana, K., Herzog, H., ... and Withers, D. J., "Critical Role for Peptide YY in Protein-Mediated Satiation and Body-Weight Regulation," Cell Metabolism, 4(3) (2006): 223-233.

12. Montmayeur, J. P., and Le Coutre, J., Fat detection: Taste, Texture, and Post Ingestive Effects, (CRC Press, 2009).

13. Wien, M. A., Sabate, J. M., Ikle, D. N., Cole, S. E., and Kandeel, F. R., "Almonds vs Complex Carbohydrates in a Weight Reduction Program," International Journal of Obesity, 27(11) (2003): 1365-1372.

14. Li, Z., Song, R., Nguyen, C., Zerlin, A., Karp, H., Naowamondhol, K., ... and Henning, S. M., "Pistachio Nuts

Reduce Triglycerides and Body Weight by Comparison to Refined Carbohydrate Snack in Obese Subjects on a 12-Week Weight Loss Program," Journal of the American College of Nutrition, 29(3) (2010): 198-203.

15. McManus, K., Antinoro, L., and Sacks, F., "A Randomized Controlled Trial of a Moderate-Fat, Low-Energy Diet Compared with a Low Fat, Low-Energy Diet for Weight Loss in Overweight Adults," International Journal of Obesity, 25(10) (2001): 1503-1511.

16. Foster, G. D., Shantz, K. L., Vander Veur, S. S., Oliver, T. L., Lent, M. R., Virus, A., ... and Gilden-Tsai, A., "A Randomized Trial of the Effects of an Almond-Enriched, Hypocaloric Diet in the Treatment of Obesity," The American Journal of Clinical Nutrition, 96(2) (2012): 249-254.

17. Pelkman, C. L., Fishell, V. K., Maddox, D. H., Pearson, T. A., Mauger, D. T., and Kris-Etherton, P. M., "Effects of Moderate-Fat (from monounsaturated fat) and Low-Fat Weight-Loss Diets on the Serum Lipid Profile in Overweight and Obese Men and Women," The American Journal of Clinical Nutrition, 79(2) (2004): 204-212.

18. Wien, M. A., Sabate, J. M., Ikle, D. N., Cole, S. E., and Kandeel, F. R., "Almonds vs Complex Carbohydrates in a Weight Reduction Program," International Journal of Obesity, 27(11) (2003):. 1365-1372.

19. Tan, S. Y., and Mattes, R. D., "Appetitive, Dietary and Health Effects of Almonds Consumed with Meals or as Snacks: a

Randomized, Controlled Trial," European Journal of Clinical Nutrition, 67(11) (2013): 1205-1214.

20. Brennan, A. M., Sweeney, L. L., Liu, X., and Mantzoros, C. S., "Walnut Consumption Increases Satiation but Has No Effect on Insulin Resistance or the Metabolic Profile over a 4-Day Period. Obesity, 18(6) (2010): 1176-1182.

21. Fraser, G. E., Bennett, H. W., Jaceldo, K. B., and Sabaté, J., "Effect on Body Weight of a Free 76 Kilojoule (320 calorie) Daily Supplement of Almonds for Six Months," Journal of the American College of Nutrition, 21(3) (2002): 275-283.

22. Alper, C. Á., & Mattes, R. D.," Effects of Chronic Peanut Consumption on Energy Balance and Hedonics," International Journal of Obesity, 26(8) (2002): 1129-1137.

23. Tan, S. Y., Dhillon, J., and Mattes, R. D., A Review of the Effects of Nuts on Appetite, Food Intake, Metabolism, and Body Weight," The American Journal ofCclinical Nutrition, 100(suppl_1) (2014): 412S-422S.

Chapter Six

1. National Center for Health Statistics US. (2019). Health, United States, 2018.

2. Sievert, K., Hussain, S. M., Page, M. J., Wang, Y., Hughes, H. J., Malek, M., and Cicuttini, F. M., "Effect of Breakfast on Weight and Energy Intake: Systematic Review and Meta-Analysis of Randomised Controlled Trials," bmj, (2019): 364.

3. Rains, T. M., Leidy, H. J., Sanoshy, K. D., Lawless, A. L., & Maki, K. C.," A Randomized, Controlled, Crossover Trial to Assess the Acute Appetitive and Metabolic Effects of Sausage and Egg-Based Convenience Breakfast Meals in Overweight Premenopausal Women," Nutrition Journal, 14(1) (2015): 1-10.

4. Leidy, H. J., and Racki, E. M. The addition of a Protein-Rich Breakfast and Its Effects on Acute Appetite Control and Food Intake in 'Breakfast-Skipping' Adolescents. International Journal of Obesity, 34(7) (2010): 1125-1133.

5. Meinert, L., Kehlet, U., and Aaslyng, M. D., "Consuming Pork Proteins at Breakfast Reduces the Feeling of Hunger Before Lunch," Appetite, 59(2) (2012): 201-203.

6. Blom, W. A., Lluch, A., Stafleu, A., Vinoy, S., Holst, J. J., Schaafsma, G., and Hendriks, H. F., "Effect of a High-Protein Breakfast on the Postprandial Ghrelin Response," The American Journal of Clinical Nutrition, 83(2) (2006):. 211-220.

7. Leidy, H. J., and Racki, E. M., "The Addition of a Protein-Rich Breakfast and its Effects on Acute Appetite Control and Food Intake in 'Breakfast-Skipping' Adolescents," International Journal of Obesity, 34(7) (2010): 1125-1133.

8. Wang, S., Yang, L., Lu, J., and Mu, Y., H:gh-Protein Breakfast Promotes Weight Loss by Suppressing Subsequent Food Intake and Regulating Appetite Hormones in Obese Chinese Adolescents," Hormone Research in Pediatrics, 83(1) (2015): 19-25.

9. Vander Wal, J. S., Gupta, A., Khosla, P., and Dhurandhar, N. V., "Egg Breakfast Enhances Weight Loss," International Journal of Obesity, 32(10) (2008): 1545-1551.

10. Taheri, S., Lin, L., Austin, D., Young, T., and Mignot, E., "Short Sleep Duration is Associated with Reduced Leptin, Elevated Ghrelin, and Increased Body Mass Index," PLoS Med, 1(3) (2004): e62.

11. Al Khatib, H. K., Harding, S. V., Darzi, J., and Pot, G. K., "The Effects of Partial Sleep Deprivation on Energy Balance: a Systematic Review and Meta-Analysis," European Journal of Clinical Nutrition," 71(5) (2017): 614-624.

12. St-Onge, M. P., Roberts, A., Shechter, A., and Choudhury, A. R.," Fiber and Saturated Fat are Associated with Sleep Arousals and Slow Wave Sleep," Journal of Clinical Sleep Medicine, 12(1) (2016): 19-24.

13. Crispim, C. A., Zimberg, I. Z., dos Reis, B. G., Diniz, R. M., Tufik, S., and de Mello, M. T., "Relationship Between Food Intake and Sleep Pattern in Healthy Individuals," Journal of Clinical Sleep Medicine, 7(6) (2011): 659-664.

Chapter Seven

1. Kaplan, H. I., and Kaplan, H. S., "The Psychosomatic Concept of Obesity," Journal of Nervous and Mental Disease, (1957)..

2. Schachter, S., "Obesity and Eating.," Science, (1968).

3. Bruch, H.," Four Decades of Eating Disorders," Handbook of Psychotherapy for Anorexia Nervosa and Bulimia, 7-18 (1985)..

4. Novick, J. S., Stewart, J. W., Wisniewski, S. R., Cook, I. A., Manev, R., Nierenberg, A. A., ... and Zisook, S., "Clinical and Demographic Features of Atypical Depression in Outpatients with Major Depressive Disorder: Preliminary Findings from STAR* D.," The Journal of Clinical Psychiatry, (2005)..

5. Simon, G. E., Von Korff, M., Saunders, K., Miglioretti, D. L., Crane, P. K., Van Belle, G., and Kessler, R. C., "Association Between Obesity and Psychiatric Disorders in the US Adult Population," Archives of General Psychiatry, 63(7) (2006): 824-830.

6. Kloiber, S., Ising, M., Reppermund, S., Horstmann, S., Dose, T., Majer, M., ... and Lucae, S., "Overweight and Obesity Affect Treatment Response in Major Depression," Biological Psychiatry, 62(4) (2007): 321-326.

7. Masheb, R. M., and Grilo, C. M., "Emotional Overeating and its Associations with Eating Disorder Psychopathology Among Overweight Patients with Binge Eating Disorder," International Journal of Eating Disorders, 39(2) (2006): 141-146.

8. Rosenbaum, D. L., and White, K. S., "The Relation of Anxiety, Depression, and Stress to Binge Eating Behavior," Journal of Health Psychology, 20(6) (2015): 887-898.

9. Heatherton, T. F., an Baumeister, R. F., "Binge Eating as Escape from Self-Awareness," Psychological Bulletin, 110(1) (1991):.86.

10. Safer, D. L., Telch, C. F., and Chen, E. Y., Dialectical Behavior Therapy for Binge Eating and Bulimia. (Guilford Press, 2009).

11. Hayes, S. C., Wilson, K. G., Gifford, E. V., Follette, V. M., and Strosahl, K., "Experiential Avoidance and Behavioral Disorders: A Functional Dimensional Approach to Diagnosis and Treatment," Journal of Consulting and Clinical Psychology, 64(6) (1996): 1152.

12. Macht, M., "How Emotions Affect Eating: A Five-Way Model," Appetite, 50(1) (2008): 1-11.

13. Sharma, S., and Fulton, S., Diet-Induced Obesity Promotes Depressive-Like Behaviour that is Associated with Neural Adaptations in Brain Reward Circuitry," International Journal of Obesity, 37(3) (2013): 382-389.

14. Singh, M., "Mood, Food, and Obesity," Frontiers in Psychology, 5 (2014): 925.

Chapter Eight

1. Donnelly, J. E., Honas, J. J., Smith, B. K., Mayo, M. S., Gibson, C. A., Sullivan, D. K., ... and Washburn, R. A., "Aerobic Exercise Alone Results in Clinically Significant Weight Loss

for Men and Women: Midwest Exercise Trial 2," Obesity, 21(3) (2013): E219-E228.

2. King, N. A., Horner, K., Hills, A. P., Byrne, N. M., Wood, R. E., Bryant, E., ... and Martins, C., "Exercise, Appetite and Weight Management: Understanding the Compensatory Responses in Eating Behaviour and How They Contribute to Variability in Exercise-Induced Weight Loss," British Journal of Sports Medicine, 46(5) (2012): 315-322.

3. Ismail, I., Keating, S. E., Baker, M. K., and Johnson, N. A., "A Systematic Review and Meta-Analysis of the Effect of Aerobic vs. Resistance Exercise Training on Visceral Fat," Obesity Reviews, 13(1) (2012): 68-91.

4. Keating, S. E., Hackett, D. A., Parker, H. M., O'Connor, H. T., Gerofi, J. A., Sainsbury, A., ... and Johnson, N. A., "Effect of Aerobic Exercise Training Dose on Liver Fat and Visceral Adiposity," Journal of Hepatology, 63(1) (2015): 174-182.

5. Børsheim, E., and Bahr, R., "Effect of Exercise Intensity, Duration and Mode on Post-Exercise Oxygen Consumption." Sports Medicine, 33(14) (2003): 1037-1060.

6. Laforgia, J., Withers, R. T., and Gore, C. J., "Effects of Exercise Intensity and Duration on the Excess Post-Exercise Oxygen Consumption," Journal of Sports Sciences, 24(12) (2006):1247-1264.

7. Broom, D. R., Batterham, R. L., King, J. A., and Stensel, D. J., "Influence of Resistance and Aerobic Exercise on Hunger,

Circulating Levels of Acylated Ghrelin, and Peptide YY in Healthy Males," American Journal of Physiology-Regulatory, Integrative and Comparative Physiology (2009).

8. Dorling, J., Broom, D. R., Burns, S. F., Clayton, D. J., Deighton, K., James, L. J., ... and Stensel, D. J., "Acute and Chronic Effects of Exercise on Appetite, Energy Intake, and Appetite-Related Hormones: the Modulating Effect of Adiposity, Sex, and Habitual Physical Activity," Nutrients, 10(9) (2018): 1140.

9. Choi, K. W., Chen, C. Y., Stein, M. B., Klimentidis, Y. C., Wang, M. J., Koenen, K. C., and Smoller, J. W., "Assessment of Bidirectional Relationships Between Physical Activity and Depression Among Adults: a 2-Sample Mendelian Randomization Study," JAMA Psychiatry, 76(4) (2019): 399-408.

Chapter Nine

1. Haff, G. G., and Triplett, N. T. (Eds.). Essentials of Strength Training and Conditioning 4th Edition. (Human Kinetics, 2015).

2. Jequier, E., and Schutz, Y., "Long-Term Measurements of Energy Expenditure in Humans Using a Respiration Chamber." The American Journal of Clinical Nutrition, 38(6) (1983): 989-998.

3. Ravussin, E., Burnand, B., Schutz, Y., and Jequier, E., "Twenty-Four-Hour Energy Expenditure and Resting Metabolic Rate in Obese, Moderately Obese, and Control Subjects." The American Journal of Clinical Nutrition, 35(3) (1982):. 566-573.

4. Zello, G. A., "Dietary Reference Intakes for the Macronutrients and Energy: Considerations for Physical Activity," Applied Physiology, Nutrition, and Metabolism, 31(1) (2006):.74-79.

5. Nelson, K. M., Weinsier, R. L., Long, C. L., and Schutz, Y., "Prediction of Resting Energy Expenditure from Fat-Free Mass and Fat Mass," The American Journal of Clinical Nutrition, 56(5) (1992): 848-856.

6. Ravussin, Eric, Stephen Lillioja, Thomas E. Anderson, Laurent Christin, and Clifton Bogardus, "Determinants of 24-Hour Energy Expenditure in Man. Methods and Results Using a Respiratory Chamber," The Journal of Clinical Investigation 78, no. 6 (1986): 1568-1578.

7. Westcott, W. L., "Resistance Training is Medicine: Effects of Strength Training on Health," Current Sports Medicine Reports, 11(4) (2012): 209-216.

8. Pratley, R., Nicklas, B., Rubin, M., Miller, J., Smith, A., Smith, M., ... and Goldberg, A., "Strength Training Increases Resting Metabolic Rate and Norepinephrine Levels in Healthy 50-to 65-Yr-Old Men," Journal of Applied Physiology, 76(1) (1994): 133-137.

9. Zurlo, F., Larson, K., Bogardus, C., and Ravussin, E., "Skeletal Muscle Metabolism is a Major Determinant of Resting Energy Expenditure," The Journal of Clinical Investigation, 86(5) (1990): 1423-1427.

10. Williamson, D. L., and Kirwan, J. P., "A Single Bout of Concentric Resistance Exercise Increases Basal Metabolic Rate 48 Hours After Exercise in Healthy 59–77-Year-Old Men," The Journals of Gerontology Series A: Biological Sciences and Medical Sciences, 52(6) (1997): M352-M355.

11. Tipton, K., and Wolfe, R. R., "Exercise, Protein Metabolism, and Muscle Growth," International Journal of Sport Nutrition and Exercise Metabolism, 11(1) (2001): 109-132.

12. Heymsfield, S. B., Gonzalez, M. C., Shen, W., Redman, L., and Thomas, D., "Weight Loss Composition is One-Fourth Fat-Free Mass: A Critical Review and Critique of This Widely Cited Rule," Obesity Reviews, 15(4) (2014): 310-321.

13. Keys, A., and Grande, F. Body, "Weight, Body Composition and Calorie Status," Modern Nutrition in Health and Disease, (1973).

14. Hunter, G. R., Byrne, N. M., Sirikul, B., Fernández, J. R., Zuckerman, P. A., Darnell, B. E., and Gower, B. A., "Resistance Training Conserves Fat-Free Mass and Resting Energy Expenditure Following Weight Loss," Obesity, 16(5) (2008): 1045-1051.

15. Feigenbaum, M. S., and Pollock, M. L., "Prescription of Resistance Training for Health and Disease," Medicine and Science in Sports and Exercise, 31(1) (1999): 38-45.

16. Schoenfeld, B. J., Contreras, B., Krieger, J., Grgic, J., Delcastillo, K., Belliard, R., and Alto, A., "Resistance Training

Volume Enhances Muscle Hypertrophy but Not Strength in Trained Men," Medicine and Science in Sports and Exercise, 51(1) (2019): 94.

Chapter Eleven

1. Decision Science News, (2014) "What size will you be after you lose weight?" Retrieved from: http://www.decisionsciencenews.com/2014/11/14/size-will-lose-weight/

Chapter Twelve

1. Haimovitz, K., and Henderlong Corpus, J., "Effects of Person Versus Process Praise on Student Motivation: Stability and Change in Emerging Adulthood," Educational Psychology, 31(5) (2011): 595-609.

Made in the USA
Middletown, DE
06 July 2021

43719326R00176